More pre-publication
REVIEWS, COMMENTARIES, EVALUATIONS . . .

"*Children's Rights: Policy and Practice* is a comprehensive review and analysis of the more salient issues related to understanding, interpreting, and implementing the legal, social, and civil rights of children and adolescents in the United States. This book documents in detail the history of how the prevailing understanding of the child influences the rights that are extended to persons of that status. The development of child advocacy and the tension created between the notions of family privacy and sanctity and state intervention are also examined. Family policy and clinical approaches to child protection and support are reviewed in the context of current legislation and research.

The second edition of this book is an important contribution to the literature on children's rights, intervention, advocacy, and protection. As with the first edition, this text is an invaluable tool for students, practitioners, researchers, and advocates. Legislation regarding children's rights is well documented and, more importantly, the accompanying theories, concepts, and practical concerns are presented in detail in accessible language. The discussion of rights is framed in the context of the major institutional settings, such as schools, day care, residential treatment, and protective services, that are charged with caring for children. Readers are provided with a 'hands-on' approach, as case studies are presented throughout. This approach is one of the real strengths of the book and why it serves the needs of both novice and experienced practitioners. In sum, this text is an excellent resource for anyone concerned about the rights of children; it is a must-read for everyone involved in the advocacy and protection of children."

Karen A. Callaghan, PhD
Professor of Sociology,
Barry University

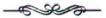

"**T**his book is essential, up-to-date reading for anyone who teaches courses that focus on family and child welfare. This edition of the book is the author's legacy to the social work profession and the field of child welfare. The comprehensive nature of this book positions it as a must-read for those students in child welfare, school social work, and family-centered practice, as well as for practitioners in a variety of human service agencies. The content and readability of the book is impressive!"

Martha J. Markward, PhD, ACSW
Associate Professor,
School of Social Work
University of Missouri

The Haworth Press
New York • London • Oxfo

Children's Rights
Policy and Practice

Second Edition

THE HAWORTH PRESS
Social Work Practice with Children and Families
Francis K. O. Yuen, DSW, ACSW
Senior Editor

Social Work Practice with Children and Families: A Family Health Approach edited by Francis K. O. Yuen

Handbook for the Treatment of Abused and Neglected Children edited by P. Forrest Talley

Homelessness in Rural America: Policy and Practice by Paul A. Rollinson and John T. Pardeck

Children's Rights: Policy and Practice, Second Edition by John T. Pardeck

Titles of Related Interest:

Using Books in Clinical Social Work Practice: A Guide to Bibliotherapy by John T. Pardeck

Reason and Rationality in Health and Human Services Delivery edited by John T. Pardeck, Charles F. Longino Jr., and John W. Murphy

Family Health Social Work Practice: A Knowledge and Skills Casebook edited by Francis K. O. Yuen, Gregory J. Skibinski, and John T. Pardeck

Disability Issues for Social Workers and Human Services Professionals in the Twenty-First Century edited by John W. Murphy and John T. Pardeck

Children's Rights
Policy and Practice

Second Edition

John T. Pardeck, PhD, LCSW

The Haworth Press
New York • London • Oxford

For more information on this book or to order, visit
http://www.haworthpress.com/store/product.asp?sku=5533

or call 1-800-HAWORTH (800-429-6784) in the United States and Canada
or (607) 722-5857 outside the United States and Canada

or contact orders@HaworthPress.com

The Haworth Press, Inc., 10 Alice Street, Binghamton, NY 13904-1580.

PUBLISHER'S NOTE
The development, preparation, and publication of this work has been undertaken with great care. However, the Publisher, employees, editors, and agents of The Haworth Press are not responsible for any errors contained herein or for consequences that may ensue from use of materials or information contained in this work. The Haworth Press is committed to the dissemination of ideas and information according to the highest standards of intellectual freedom and the free exchange of ideas. Statements made and opinions expressed in this publication do not necessarily reflect the views of the Publisher, Directors, management, or staff of The Haworth Press, Inc., or an endorsement by them.

Cover design by Christie R. Peterson.

Library of Congress Cataloging-in-Publication Data

Pardeck, John T.
    Children's rights : policy and practice / John T. Pardeck.— 2nd ed.
      p. cm.
    Includes bibliographical references and index.
    ISBN-13: 978-0-7890-2811-2 (hard : alk. paper)
    ISBN-10: 0-7890-2811-5 (hard : alk. paper)
    ISBN-13: 978-0-7890-2812-9 (soft : alk. paper)
    ISBN-10: 0-7890-2812-3 (soft : alk. paper)
    1. Children's rights—United States. 2. Child welfare—United States. 3. Social work with children—United States. 4. Children—Legal status, laws, etc.—United States. I. Title.
HQ789.P295 2005
362.7'0973—dc22
                                                      2005016519

In Memory

A TIRELESS ADVOCATE FOR HUMAN RIGHTS, Dr. John Terry Pardeck died on November 6, 2004. He valiantly fought his own battle against cancer for eighteen months, the second in his lifetime, while continuing to share as much of his knowledge and wisdom as possible through publications still coming to press at this time.

Dr. Pardeck put tremendous effort into any endeavor. His enthusiasm for teaching and serving as a mentor for students inspired many to go forth into the world as social workers. Dr. Pardeck was passionate about research and publications; his thirty books and over 130 journal articles attest to that. He served on many journal editorial boards and eventually saw the need to give birth to a journal of his own. Yet Dr. Pardeck did not limit his skills to the academic world. He provided leadership to many statewide boards and organizations dealing with advocacy, social justice, and human civil rights.

Known as Terry to friends and family, he was also a champion of their rights. Terry once made sure he got on the board of a social service agency, where he felt his wife and her colleagues were not being treated fairly, and helped steer the agency toward better practices. According to one of his sons, Terry tried to improve society by fighting for individuals, his own sons included. He spent many hours following the chain of command within a school district and at the state level to ensure that his sons were included in programs they each qualified for. Terry's other son recalls that he worked very, very hard, not just at his job but at home with his family. As soon as he found something was not right and needed change, he would do everything in his power to make it right, whether it be something small, such as writing a letter, or something much more involved, such as running for school board.

Many lives, both professionally and personally, were touched by Dr. John Terry Pardeck. We will all miss his passion to help those who could not help themselves and his respect for all human beings. He definitely left the world better than he found it. We will strive to carry on your legacy, Terry!

Jean A. Musick Pardeck
Jonathan T. Pardeck
James K. Pardeck

This book is dedicated to my wife, Jean A. Pardeck

CONTENTS

ABOUT THE AUTHOR

John T. Pardeck, PhD, was Emeritus Professor of Social Work in the School of Social Work at Southwest Missouri State University in Springfield, Missouri. Prior to this position, he was Chair of the Department of Social Work at Southeast Missouri State University. Dr. Pardeck was widely known throughout the state as an advocate for persons with disabilities and for interpreting the Americans with Disabilities Act to both private and public sector organizations.

Dr. Pardeck wrote more than 130 articles that have been published in professional and academic journals and authored, co-authored, edited, or co-edited thirty books, including *Using Books in Clinical Social Work Practice*; *Reason and Rationality in Health and Human Services Delivery*; *Postmodernism, Religion, and the Future of Social Work*; and *Social Work: Seeking Relevancy in the Twenty-First Century* (all published by The Haworth Press, Inc.). He served on the boards of several statewide social service organizations as well as on the editorial boards of several journals. He was Editor of the *Journal of Social Work Education in Disability and Rehabilitation* and Senior Editor of two Haworth Social Work Practice Press book series—Social Work Practice with Children and Families and Social Work in Disability and Rehabilitation. Dr. Pardeck passed away in November 2004.

Foreword

Children's Rights: Policy and Practice describes the most significant laws and policies in the United States that protect and nurture children. It gives advocacy tools to families and professionals in their inevitable battles for fair treatment of children. The Americans with Disabilities Act (ADA), Individuals with Disabilities Education Act (IDEA), various child abuse and neglect laws, and others are building blocks waiting for a future structure, a "national family policy" that would nurture and support children and families rather than prod, fix, or punish them—the current political fashion in child and family welfare.

Children's rights have their modern incarnation in the freedom movements of the 1960s, which included racial minorities, women, and other oppressed people. In that blazing, creative moment, even the poor, most of whom were children, were "discovered" and promised a "war on poverty" to end the dreadful waste of human potential that is still called "virtue" in America's political culture. *Children's Rights* explains the historical roots of America's willful neglect of its poor and vulnerable people, roots marked by a Calvinistic attitude that blames the poor—in essence blaming the children—for their plight and views them as individual fix-it projects rather than casualties of the social ecology of America. It cites the U.S. Constitution, which defines the relationship of government to individuals, not the government to families and children, as an explanation and manifestation of the country's boundless individualism, indifferent to the needs of others.

The ADA, IDEA, child welfare, and case law give tools to skillful advocates in an indifferent culture that sometimes responds to dedicated pounding. However, give the devil his due—those who are for less government, regulation, taxation, and services for people who need them dominate and have squeezed the juice out of community responsibility, compassion, and generosity administered by government.

For example, *Children's Rights* instructs conscientious social workers on how to investigate and intervene in child abuse cases and on how to evaluate families and obtain for them the most appropriate services to restore them to wholeness. However, it does not mention the exhaustion of a social worker with 200 cases or the waiting lists for therapeutic child care or the starvation wages for service workers that burn the idealism and creative energy out of them. Starving human services for resources is the most common and effective way to nullify humane laws passed in a "weak" moment.

Children's Rights advocates for an "ecological perspective" to assess and treat families under pressure, an approach that "stresses the relationship between organisms and their social environment" (Parkdeck, 1996, p. 63). A family's problems, in other words, are the sum of its individual personalities, idiosyncrasies, relationships, and the cultural ocean in which it swims. How much of the vicious child abuse or domestic violence, for example, would be alleviated by jobs with a living wage rather than repair through psychotherapy or punishment through prison?

As a professional advocate for social justice in Missouri's oldest citizens' action organization, I have had a fair sampling of experiences, successes, and failures with Missouri's state government and legislature. Yet I learned something from *Children's Rights*: a better grasp of the tools available to advocate for children, a vocabulary for describing and arguing for more humane public policies toward children, and some much-needed cautions about respecting the humanity of the benighted other and otherwise maintaining one's sense of humor and equanimity—even when the other guy's lawyer is "cutting you a new one" in cross-examination.

Thanks to John Pardeck for another substantial contribution to the intellectual life of hard-pressed idealists and others on the endangered species list.

Peter De Simone
Executive Director
Missouri Association for Social Welfare

Preface

The second edition of *Children's Rights: Policy and Practice* was inspired by the author's work with children and their families throughout his professional career in the field of social work. He has worked as a protective services worker, as a college professor, as a guardian ad litem, as a member of several child protection teams, and as a trainer of Court Appointed Special Advocates (CASA) volunteers and foster parents. From these experiences, the author has written a second edition of this book that will be useful for those who are involved in the children's rights movement in various capacities, including academicians, child welfare workers, attorneys, volunteers, parents, and students majoring in various disciplines in the human services, including social work.

The second edition of *Children's Rights: Policy and Practice* includes new materials in the following areas:

- An update on new rulings of the Americans with Disabilities Act (ADA) that have implications for children's rights.
- Legal case studies that have relevance for children's rights. These case studies can be used as teaching tools in the classroom.
- An overview and analysis of the new No Child Left Behind Act and the implications of the act on children's rights.
- An analysis of children's rights and school violence.
- An expanded discussion on practice interventions focusing on various approaches for helping children adjust to substitute care.
- Expanded discussion on advocacy and children's rights. Particular emphasis is placed on legal case studies as a tool for enhancing children's rights.

Chapter 1 introduces the reader to the children's rights movement that largely emerged in the 1960s. Since the 1960s, a number of significant court rulings and important national legislation have increased the rights of children. Notable court rulings discussed in Chapter 1 are *In re Gault* (1967) and *Kent v. United States* (1966). These court rulings resulted in new protections for children in the juvenile justice system. Since the 1970s, national legislation has been enacted protecting children from abuse and neglect; additional comprehensive legislation has been enacted aimed at improving the services for children placed in foster care and adoption. Specifically, the Congress passed the Child Abuse Prevention and Treatment Act (CAPTA) in 1974; the purpose of this policy was to prevent and treat child abuse. The Adoption Assistance and Child Welfare Act of 1980 was enacted in order to improve the lives of children placed in adoption and foster care. The reader will note that a detailed discussion is offered in Chapter 1 on the effect of adoption and foster care placement on children; the research on this topic clearly suggests that placement in care has a number of psychological and social consequences for children. Chapter 1 concludes by showing how one of the most basic rights that children are entitled to, freedom from poverty, is heavily influenced by race and geographical area. It is suggested that strong legislation aimed at improving the lives of children living in families with incomes below the poverty level must be passed.

Chapter 2 focuses on the rights of parents and their children. It is suggested that the rights of each party may at times conflict. When this occurs the court system must decide whose rights will prevail, the child or his or her parents. However, it must be noted that when parents fail at their parenting obligations, it is important for the state to intervene in family life. The chapter offers a healthy discussion on the problems related to state intervention into family life, stressing that even though the law may be vague in this area, some children must be removed from their biological families for their own protection. It is noted in Chapter 2 that in general, the rights of parents outweigh those of children. The answer to why such is the case can be partially found in the child-development literature. Specifically, Chapter 2 emphasizes that children do not have the cognitive and intellectual capacity to make informed decisions about their lives until reaching a certain age. Chapter 2 offers numerous Supreme Court rulings that better define the rights of parents, children, and government. Chapter 2 also includes a debate between the child liberationists and child protectionists concerning the age at which children should be allowed to make decisions that have important consequences for their lives.

Chapter 3 presents the rights of children in schools. Given the dramatic increase in legislation aimed at children with disabilities in the school system, much of this chapter focuses on the newfound rights of special needs children. The chapter offers a detailed discussion on the Individuals with Disabilities Educational Act (IDEA) and the Americans with Disabilities Act (ADA) of 1990. Recent ADA rulings that have implications for children's rights are covered, as well as revisions in IDEA. Also offered is an overview and analysis of the No Child Left Behind Act and its implications for children's rights. The rights of all children in schools, including those with special needs, are discussed in this chapter. It must be recognized, however, that states vary greatly on the rights that protect all children in schools. Given this situation, the discussion focuses on the rights of children in schools related to issues such as freedom of expression and speech, censorship, and school safety versus privacy. Particular emphasis is placed on the perceived problem of school violence. What is suggested in Chapter 3 is that children lose most of their constitutional rights at the schoolhouse door. It is concluded in the chapter that children will probably continue to lose basic rights, such as a right to privacy, in the school setting.

The ADA has not only affected schools but also day care programs. The reader will find that Chapter 4 covers the requirements mandated by the ADA for children with disabilities in day care programs. As with public education, states vary greatly on the rights of all children in day care settings. The state agency that regulates day care programs is typically the department of social services. Throughout the United States, tremendous variability exists in the educational requirements of day care staff, space requirements for day care providers, and general licensing requirements for operating day care programs. What this means is that the basic rights children are entitled to in day care programs largely depend on the state where the child lives. The author stresses, however, that the ADA requirements must be followed by all day care providers regardless of whether they are public or private. The discussion of these requirements should prove helpful to those working in day care programs, as well as those training for careers in child care and development. Finally, a detailed discussion is offered on the impact of day care on children and the policy implications of current day care policy in the United States.

Chapter 5 explores the rights of children in residential settings. Given the fact that placement in residential treatment is often involuntary, protecting the rights of children in such settings is critical. The chapter offers the reader a number of ethical dilemmas that practitioners often face when working with children in residential treatment. The chapter stresses that since treatment teams are composed of various professionals, they must be sure to work as a team in order to ensure children in residential treatment receive the services they need.

Chapter 6 presents the role and function of protective services in the child welfare system. Protective services provide help for families at risk and are largely aimed at children who have been abused and neglected. Abuse and neglect are the predominant reasons why children enter the foster care system. The chapter offers a number of theories attempting to explain the causes of abuse and neglect and concludes that an ecological perspective appears to provide the most useful explanation for why certain families are at greater risk for child maltreatment than others. Chapter 6 emphasizes the need for more rigorous research in the area of child maltreatment and suggests that an ecological approach that includes family therapy as a core treatment modality offers the most useful strategy for working with families at risk. The chapter concludes with the process used by protective services to provide help to families at risk. A recent study is presented that reports a relationship between child maltreatment and homelessness, an issue that has obvious implications for the rights of children.

Advocacy is a critical policy and practice activity for practitioners involved in the children's rights movement. Chapter 7 argues that advocacy should be conducted at two different levels: case advocacy and cause advocacy. Case advocacy is used when advocating for an individual child. Cause advocacy includes advocating for a collective group of children. The chapter offers advocacy skills that parents should find useful for helping them advocate for the rights of their children in various settings. Parents of special needs children should find these skills to be particularly helpful when confronted with school systems that do not offer the services their children need. The chapter also includes advocacy techniques for professionals, illustrating them through a case example. Chapter 7 stresses that a number of laws are in place, including laws protecting special needs children, which are not being implemented by schools and other institutions.

Case and cause advocacy activities are often called for when organizations do not comply with these laws. A detailed analysis of using litigation as an advocacy strategy is offered, along with a number of legal rulings illustrating the power of this form of advocacy for ensuring the rights of children.

The final chapter of the book analyzes the implications of children's rights on policy and practice. The chapter suggests that one of the greatest threats to children's rights is poverty. Children who live below the poverty level are often denied a right to quality health care, proper nutrition, adequate housing, and quality schools. The author calls for a comprehensive family policy aimed at helping all families in the United States. Comprehensive family policy would have a dramatic impact on the ecosystems that influence the lives of families and their children. Presently family policy in the United States is fragmented and underdeveloped. Comprehensive family policy would greatly reduce the need for protective services because so many of the problems that bring families to the attention of protective services would be eliminated through a comprehensive national family policy. The chapter concludes with an emerging practice orientation, family health, that includes expanded effective strategies for assessing and treating children in substitute care; furthermore, practitioners in the field of social work and related disciplines are finding the family health approach to be very useful for working with children and families. Family health effectively integrates policy with practice; this means that intervention takes place at both the micro and macro levels. Protecting the rights of children is a critical philosophical grounding for practitioners using the family health approach to practice.

Chapter 1

The Children's Rights Movement

According to Hawes (1991), the modern children's rights movement emerged in the 1960s. Since that time there have been many developments in this movement. These include greater awareness of child maltreatment, the passage of national legislation aimed at improving the lives of children, significant court rulings, and the emergence of a number of child advocacy groups. Even with these important changes, the following research findings suggest that children continue to live under less-than-ideal conditions in the United States:

1. The decreasing number of children in the United States will result in less legislative attention aimed at their needs. Research reports that in 1960 children accounted for 36 percent of all Americans; in 1990 they were 26 percent, and by 2010 only 23 percent of the population will be children (U.S. Department of Commerce, Bureau of the Census, 1989, 1990).
2. Over the past thirty years, a rapidly rising divorce rate and an increase in out-of-wedlock childbearing has dramatically increased the numbers of children living with one parent (Chung and Pardeck, 1997).
3. One of the most relevant changes over the past several decades has been the increasing numbers of mothers entering the workforce. For example, between 1970 and 1990, the proportion of mothers with children under age six who were working or looking for work rose from 32 percent to 58 percent. This number has increased to over 80 percent of women with children between the ages of six and thirteen who were working or looking for work (Chung and Pardeck, 1997).
4. Children today are the poorest Americans; one in four children lives in a family below the poverty level (Chung and Pardeck, 1997).

5. Forty-three million Americans, including millions of children under age eighteen, have no health insurance coverage. This number continues to increase despite efforts made even with the various attempts by state governments to certify more children for Medicaid (Chung and Pardeck, 1997).
6. One in four adolescents engages in some form of behavior that leads to serious, long-term problems (Carnegie Council on Adolescent Development, 1989). For example, in the 1980s, approximately 1 million teenage girls became pregnant each year; half of them give birth. Only recently has the number of teenage pregnancies begun to drop (Chung and Pardeck, 1997).
7. Approximately 500,000 young people drop out of school each year (Kaufman and Frase, 1990).
8. Since 1981, we have seen an 80 percent rise in the proportion of children receiving psychological assistance annually. This number continues to increase (Chung and Pardeck, 1997).

In most industrialized nations, children have a right to health care as well as other social services (Aldrich and Associates, 1976; Berger and Neuhaus, 1977; and Karger and Stoesz, 2001). This is not the case in the United States (Cherlin, 1988; Kain-Caudle, 1973; Kamerman and Kahn, 1976; Keniston and The Carnegie Council on Children, 1977; National Commission on Children, 1991; Schorr, 1968; · Tropman, 1985; Pardeck, 1990). Within American society, the infant mortality rates in some areas are higher than in many third world countries. This high infant mortality rate can be traced directly to poverty. Consequently, the most basic right of any child, the right to life itself, is dependent on the economic status of his or her parents, and that in turn varies by race and geographical region (Hawes, 1991; Zill and Schoenborn, 1990).

Even though many children in the United States are deprived of basic economic supports (Chung and Pardeck, 1997; O'Hare et al., 1990; Rice, 1977), great efforts have been made in improving their civil rights. The civil rights movement of the 1960s, in particular, created an environment resulting in significant changes for not only minorities but also children. Specifically, court rulings during the 1960s endorsed the notion that children have rights independent of their parents. Basic constitutional guarantees were extended to young people, including the right to due process at the jurisdictional phase in delinquency proceedings, such as the right to legal counsel and the right to confront and cross examine witnesses (Hawes, 1991).

The constitutionalization of children's rights has provided a framework for litigation against agencies providing child welfare services. The courts also have held that in loco parentis status cannot be used as a strategy to negate a child's legal rights. Specifically, children who are in custody for a crime have important constitutional protections, including the right to contest confinement, to be free of arbitrary punishment, and to receive treatment (McGowan and Meezan, 1983).

Of great significance in the area of child welfare, children placed in substitute care have a right to permanency in the most familylike setting. This right emerged from the Adoption Assistance and Child Welfare Act of 1980. The philosophical grounding to the right of permanency evolved from Goldstein, Freud, and Solnit's (1973) book *Beyond the Best Interests of the Child*. In their work, they emphasize the importance of the "psychological parent" to the child; this notion has had a profound impact on child welfare policy and practices.

The Adoption Assistance and Child Welfare Act of 1980 requires that the child's biological parents participate in the permanent plan and that the plan be subject to review on a periodic basis. The permanent plan is guided by the following principles (Kadushin and Martin, 1988):

1. The birth family has the capacity to change and thereby provide healthy continuity in which the child can develop.
2. It is the child welfare system's role to work collaboratively with the family in developing and implementing a permanent plan.
3. Plans are designed to assure the continuity of the child's development. Continuity is reflected by the alternatives of the child residing in his or her own home, a relative's home, or an adoptive home.
4. Services are time-limited, with worker-family-defined expectations and outcomes.
5. Although the reason for intervention with the family is to assure the safety of the child, the focus of the services is to better prepare the parents to meet the child's needs.
6. If the child is in alternative care, the caregivers must be part of the therapeutic process. One of the worker's roles is to problem solve with the caregivers to help them fulfill their role with the child.

Permanency planning minimizes the tendency to simply react to crisis. It provides a framework for agencies responding to children and families as they come to the child welfare system's attention.

One of the more critical goals of the permanency plan is to return children to their biological parents. If the child is not able to return to his or her biological parents, adoption is seen as the second most desirable outcome. The least-ideal outcome of the permanency plan is long-term, stable foster care.

CHILD MALTREATMENT AND CHILDREN'S RIGHTS

The passage of the Child Abuse Prevention and Treatment Act (CAPTA) of 1974 has helped to protect children from abuse and neglect. This law requires states to meet basic federal standards on custody provisions, which include granting state child welfare agencies the power to remove children from families for up to three days if an agency believes the child is at risk. Prior to the passage of CAPTA, states had variable standards in place for protecting children from maltreatment.

In the 1960s and 1970s, social scientists began to study the rates and causes of child abuse and neglect in the United States (Helfer and Kempe, 1968; Gil, 1970). This research was used by Congress as the basis for the passage of CAPTA. What studies generally confirmed is that it is difficult to differentiate between abusing and non-abusing families (Hawes, 1991). The following lists some of the most critical findings from this research (Hawes, 1991):

1. Unemployment of fathers is correlated with higher rates of child abuse.
2. Isolated and large families have a greater tendency to be abusive.
3. The willingness of authoritarian figures to endorse physical punishment is associated with higher rates of abuse.

There was little opposition to the passage of CAPTA. However, as the law was implemented critics did emerge. One critic, Robert Mnookin (1973), suggested that the new law resulted in a flood of unfounded child abuse and neglect reports that already overwhelmed the limited resources of protective services agencies. Mnookin concluded that the lack of resources resulted in these agencies being less able to protect children in real danger.

Mnookin (1979) also argued that the standards under the 1974 act were vague and administered by a poorly functioning child welfare bureaucratic system. A common practice was to remove children from their families and place them in foster care. Most removals were because the parent's supervision was inadequate, the mother was thought to be emotionally ill, or because of the child's behavioral problems (Hawes, 1991). Mnookin concluded that cases of intentional abuse were in the distinct minority. Mnookin (1979) was particularly opposed to the "best interest of the child" standard because judges often had incomplete information about the child and his or her parents. Judges also had great latitude in deciding what the best interest of a child should be. Mnookin (1979) concluded:

> As long as the best interest standard or some equally broad standard is used, it seems inevitable that petitions will be filed and neglect cases will be decided without any clear articulation or consistent application of the behavioral or moral premises on which the decision is based. (p. 210)

Not only was Mnookin concerned about the placement of children in foster care but also the impact of substitute care in general on children.

Goldstein, Freud, and Solnit (1973) helped to resolve some of Mnookin's concerns in their work. They concluded that children need a safe and emotionally consistent environment. To achieve this goal, they recommended the following guidelines:

1. Placement decisions should enhance the child's need for continuity of relationships.
2. Placement decisions should reflect the child's sense of time, not the adult's.
3. Child placement decisions must take into account the law's incapacity to supervise interpersonal relationships and the limits of current knowledge to make long-term predictions about human behavior.
4. Placements should provide the least detrimental alternative available for safeguarding the child's development.
5. The child in any contested placement should have full-party status and must be represented by legal counsel.

As mentioned previously, the important work of Goldstein, Freud, and Solnit (1973) served as the basis upon which the Adoption Assistance and Child Welfare Act of 1980 was grounded. Each of the previous guidelines was built into this law.

Even though national policies have been enacted to free children from abuse and neglect, maltreatment continues to be a major social problem. It is estimated that at least 1.6 million cases of abuse and neglect occur each year. Child abuse is also a major cause of death of children in the United States; it is estimated that 4,000 children die each year from abuse (Court Appointed Special Advocates, 1996).

Several hypotheses attempting to explain the causes of maltreatment have been advanced by researchers (Helfer and Kempe, 1968; Gil, 1970). Research findings suggest that child abuse is correlated with rigid, authoritarian, isolated family systems. These families are often experiencing marital, financial, or parent-child problems and typically lack resources and skills to cope with everyday problems. Poverty and unemployment add to the stress of these family systems.

Three kinds of child abuse have been identified: these include psychological, physical, and sexual abuse. The following describes each of these forms of maltreatment (Court Appointed Special Advocates, 1996):

1. Psychological abuse includes threatening, disparaging remarks by a caregiver or other adult.
2. Physical abuse includes commissive actions or a pattern of commissive actions on the part of a caregiver that results in injury to the child.
3. Child sexual abuse involves sexual actions involving a child in any way. This behavior may be performed by an individual other than the caregiver, with or without the caregiver's knowledge.

All of these actions have significant long-term effects on children. Children have a basic human right to be free of all forms of abuse.

Neglect is also a form of child maltreatment. Neglect involves omissive actions or a pattern of omissive actions on the part of the caregiver. These actions result in physical, educational, social, and psychological delays. A number of researchers strongly suggest that neglect may have a more profound impact on children than other forms of maltreatment (Westman, 1991).

Children who are maltreated are often placed in the foster care system (Karger and Stoesz, 2001). At present, approximately 600,000 children are in this system (Karger and Stoesz, 2001). The Adoption Assistance and Child Welfare Act of 1980 was supposed to lower the number of children in foster care; the law has not accomplished this goal (Westman, 1991). The following discussion focuses on the foster care and adoption system. Child advocates must understand issues related to foster care and adoption in order to improve their effectiveness when working with children in these kinds of placements. Much of the children's rights movement has been aimed at improving the lives of children who have been placed in foster care and adoptive families.

FOSTER CARE AND ADOPTION

Foster care is defined as any living arrangement in which children live with people who act as substitute parents. The child welfare system in the United States was originally designed to provide temporary care for children who were maltreated or orphaned. These problems continue to be major causes of placement (Pardeck and Pardeck, 1987, 1998).

Children placed in foster care typically experience feelings of separation and loss regarding their biological parents. Placement in substitute care is often stressful and involves emotional pain. Long-term foster care is especially problematic because children may spend long periods of time in the foster care system with frequent moving from one foster home to another, and thus lack a sense of permanency (Pardeck and Pardeck, 1998).

Adoption is the treatment goal for many children in foster care. Historically, adoption services were designed to benefit parents, both biological and adoptive. Adults wanted children to continue a family name and inherit property, or they simply wanted a child to fill emotional needs. During the first half of the 1900s, the fitness of the baby and its similarity to the adoptive parents were the main concerns of child welfare workers. Unmarried girls also wanted to hide their pregnancies from the world to avoid shame; this meant that many babies coming into the world needed adoptive homes. Adoption agencies could take great care in matching the physical characteristics and other factors of biological and adoptive parents (Pardeck and Pardeck, 1998).

With the increasing use of birth control and the availability of abortion, the need for adoption has decreased. Society has become generally more accepting of single mothers, and improvements in child care facilities now free women to work outside the home and support their children financially. These developments have changed the adoption process for both adoptive parents and children. Many homes for expectant mothers that once had large adoption programs now concentrate on helping young girls keep and care for their children. The result has been fewer babies available for adoption (Pardeck and Pardeck, 1998).

Foster Care

In 1990 approximately 600,000 children were in foster care. A decade earlier, half this number were in care. This increase in numbers was attributed to the growing awareness of child abuse and neglect, as well as to the numerous problems facing families in modern society. Some of the critical concerns facing the foster care system are the increasing numbers of children entering the system and the tendency for children to experience multiple placements (Pardeck and Pardeck, 1998).

In the United States, a great deal is known about the foster care system and the unique problems facing foster children. Some of these are as follows (Downs et al., 2004):

1. Children in foster care come from all walks of life; however, there is a tendency for children in the system to be poor and from minority groups.
2. The average stay in care is about three and one-half years. Unfortunately, biological families often do not have access to quality social services while their children are in foster care.
3. Children in foster care often have parental visitation as part of their permanency plans. Most courts insist on visitation between foster children and biological parents as an intrinsic part of treatment.

4. The goal is to return foster children to their biological parents. When this is not feasible, the child should be placed for adoption. Nationally, approximately 150,000 children are available for adoption.
5. Nearly 40 percent of the children in care are thirteen years old or older.
6. Approximately 85 percent of the children in foster care have been maltreated.
7. The number of children spending their entire childhood in substitute care is close to seven percent.
8. Over 25 percent of children in foster care have experienced placement in three or more foster homes.

Children placed in foster care have a unique set of problems not faced by most children. Given these issues, foster parents as well as professionals working with foster children need varied and creative approaches to help children cope with moving into foster care placement (Pardeck and Pardeck, 1998).

Children who enter foster care often experience a series of stages in their reaction to being separated from their parents. They may wonder, for example, "Why has this happened to me?" They often feel that what has happened to them is surely a mistake. During the first several days of placement in care, many children lose their appetites, have nightmares, and experience other problems. This is part of the shock associated with separation from their parents. Some children behave very well during the first few days or weeks of placement; this phase is often short-term, and problem behaviors begin to emerge a few weeks after placement (Pardeck and Pardeck, 1998).

The second stage of the child's reaction to placement is protest. Children may do everything possible to irritate their foster parents and other adults, such as teachers, with the hope that they will be returned to their biological parents. Foster children are at times hostile toward children from intact families (Pardeck and Pardeck, 1998).

Experiencing anger after moving into foster placement is typical of foster children. It is helpful to show the child that he or she is not alone and to help the child express his or her anger in socially acceptable ways. By doing so, the child will not spend energy in hiding his or her feelings or acting them out in socially unacceptable ways (Pardeck and Pardeck, 1998).

Stage three is the time of despair. When a child gives up fighting the placement, sadness and depression increase. Many children experience developmental regression and appear to want some kind of love and comfort from their foster parents. However, when comfort is offered by the foster parent, the child may resist (Pardeck and Pardeck, 1998).

The last stage is the adjustment phase. Even though the child may never fully emotionally recover from the separation from his or her biological parents, he or she gradually adjusts to placement in care. In other words, the child accepts the reality of being placed in foster care (Pardeck and Pardeck, 1998).

Adoption

Biological family relationships begin at birth. Also, society recognizes clearly defined, socially supported entitlements for parents and children in biological families. Parents, through conception and birth, are "entitled" by society and law to be parents of a child. This results in a sense of belonging and bonding between children and their biological families (Pardeck and Pardeck, 1998).

The process of building families through adoption is far different. Adoption is more accurately described as an event similar to marriage. Marriage is not a biological event; rather, it is a legal procedure for joining two people into a family unit (Pardeck and Pardeck, 1998). Hartman (1984) concludes that marriage in a certain sense is an excellent metaphor for adoption. Adoption, like marriage, involves a process of building attachment that takes place over time. It begins when a family is approved by an agency for adoption and continues through to the placement of a child and even after placement (Pardeck and Pardeck, 1998).

As most adoptive parents come to realize, overcoming separation and building attachment with an adopted child is a difficult process. Even though adoptive parents hope a child will love them the same as his or her biological parents, love and bonding takes time. If adoptive parents are not sensitive to this issue, problems emerge not only for the adoptive parents but also for the child (Pardeck and Pardeck, 1998). Given the unique problems that are likely to occur during the adoption process, adoptive parents need support in dealing with the complexities of this process.

When children move into an adoptive home, a number of critical events occur. First, the child must begin to realize that he or she will not be returning to his or her biological parents. Even if the child has been in extended foster care, the child may continue to harbor the fantasy of returning to his or her biological family. Adoptive parents must help the child move through this fantasy; it will not be given up easily. Gradually, the fantasy will be abandoned by the child, often resulting in the child entering a stage of mourning for his or her biological parents. If this stage occurs, the child will need help in expressing anger and other feelings when reminiscing about the past and in realizing that he or she will not return to his or her biological family. Open and truthful discussion of the child's past is the most effective approach; denial and secrecy by adoptive parents can damage the child's social and emotional functioning (Pardeck and Pardeck, 1998).

Another critical aspect of the adoption process is helping the child gain self-awareness and knowledge about the past. An adopted child develops a greater sense of continuity with the past and present if he or she has knowledge about biological parents and other significant people who shared the past. This process will help the child give up fantasies about the past and clarify his or her sense of self as a person with continuity and connectedness with the adoptive family (Pardeck and Pardeck, 1998).

Once the child is placed in adoptive care, fantasies of returning to the biological family may continue and the need to connect to the past continues to be an important emotional factor. Adoptive parents should realize that children, especially those who have been abused or neglected or who are older, may be fearful, angry, and anticipating another rejection (Pardeck and Pardeck, 1998).

The first week of the adoption may go smoothly; this period of tranquility is often artificial because the child has not yet bonded with his or her adoptive family. The "honeymoon" often ends when the adoptive child begins feeling stirrings of caring and longing for biological parents. The child may even fight bonding with the adoptive family because he or she is frightened of another rejection by significant others. This tumultuous time can be reframed, however, as an indication that the child is beginning to care about his or her adoptive family. The greater the child's resistance to bonding and attachment to the adoptive family, the greater the temptation may be for the child to become a part of the adoptive family. Such a time period is difficult for the child and the adoptive parents (Pardeck and Pardeck, 1998).

The numerous issues that are likely to occur during the adoption process mean that parents need help and support in dealing with the complexities. For the child, much of what is taking place is beyond his or her control. The impact of adoption on the child is dramatic and clearly affects the child's identity and total psychological well-being. Adoptive children often search for their biological parents well into adulthood (Pardeck and Pardeck, 1998).

WELFARE REFORM AND CHILDREN'S RIGHTS

The Personal Responsibility and Work Opportunity Reconciliation Act of 1996 (HR 3734) is a dramatic departure from welfare policy since the 1930s. This legislation has had a serious consequence for the rights of children of low-income families because it no longer is an entitlement program. A major provision of HR 3734 is to move welfare policy and programs from the federal level to the state and local levels. Even though the verdict is not yet in on HR 3734, it does not appear to be a child- or family-friendly policy (Pardeck, 2002). The major provisions of HR 3734 include the following:

1. The Aid to Families with Dependent Children (AFDC) program is replaced by the Temporary Assistance for Needy Families (TANF) program. State and local governments administer TANF.
2. Under TANF, states receive a block grant that has a monetary cap. States have great discretion in how they spend the TANF money. However, when the block grant is spent, states are not entitled to additional federal funds. A contingency fund is established to help states that spend in excess of their block grant amounts; this funding is only available under limited conditions, specifically during times of high unemployment.
3. Adults who receive cash benefits are required to work or participate in a state-designed work program after two years; if they do not participate, they are ineligible for benefits. HR 3734 mandates that one individual in a household must work at least thirty hours a week.

4. States are supposed to have at least 50 percent of their total single-parent welfare cases employed. States that do not meet this requirement will have their block grants reduced by 5 percent each year until they reach this goal.
5. States can sanction clients who fail to meet the work requirement through reduction or termination of benefits.
6. Payments to recipients using federal funds must end after a maximum of five years; clients must be self-supporting at that time.
7. Food Stamps are cut out for persons between the ages of eighteen and fifty years.
8. Under HR 3734, children with disabilities can be declared ineligible for Supplemental Security Income (SSI).
9. For the first five years of residence, persons immigrating to the United States since the passage of HR 3734 are ineligible for most means-tested government programs, including TANF, Food Stamps, and Medicaid.
10. Illegal aliens are ineligible for all means-tested programs.

Given the discretion that states have in implementing HR 3734, this law appears to be less than supportive of families and may further fragment family programs. HR 3734 creates fifty distinct and different welfare states within the United States. The real meaning of HR 3734 is that it has contributed to greater uncertainty for families and does not appear to promote family functioning (Pardeck, 2002).

Using the state of Missouri as an illustration of how HR 3734 affects individuals and families has been noted by Pardeck (2002):

1. No poor child or family in Missouri is assured of economic assistance. TANF is a block grant, not a program.
2. The block grants under HR 3734 are frozen when Missouri experiences economic downturn; only a limited amount of federal help is available under HR 3734.
3. The maximum time period a family can receive TANF in Missouri is five years; no one knows what happens to needy families after the five-year time period.
4. The grant to a family of three under TANF is $292.00 per month, an amount significantly below the poverty level.

5. Medicaid eligibility and receipt of aid under TANF are delinked; families receiving ADFC were automatically eligible for Medicaid.
6. Unemployed, employable adults not raising children are limited to three months of Food Stamps in a three-year time period—over 24,000 people have lost their Food Stamps eligibility because of this rule.
7. Legal immigrants and their families are denied Food Stamps and SSI in Missouri.
8. In Missouri over 7,000 children with disabilities have lost SSI benefits.

HR 3734 has had a negative impact on needy children and families in Missouri. It has had a similar impact in other states. HR 3734 reflects the tradition in the United States of underdeveloped family policy that results in millions of children and families having inadequate health care, social services, and economic supports. HR 3734 is clearly a major setback for the rights of children.

LITIGATION AND CHILDREN'S RIGHTS

The first case to reach the Supreme Court that focused on the juvenile court was *Kent v. United States* (1966). Morris A. Kent, a sixteen-year-old child, was charged with robbery and rape. He was detained without a hearing; his case was consequently moved to criminal court. Kent's lawyer questioned whether or not the juvenile court could conduct such legal actions without a hearing; the Supreme Court ruled that Kent was entitled to a hearing. This case was significant because it provided juveniles with critical procedural rights in the juvenile court system.

In re Gault (1967) was a second case that brought about significant changes in the juvenile justice system. Gerald Gault, a fifteen-year-old boy, was charged with making obscene phone calls. A juvenile court hearing was held; following the hearing Gault was sentenced to Arizona's state industrial school until he reached the age of twenty-one. Gault's attorney, in his appeal to the Arizona Supreme Court, argued that his client's procedural rights were violated. The Arizona Supreme Court disagreed; the case ultimately reached the U.S. Supreme Court, which concluded that the juvenile court violated Gault's procedural rights by denying him due process. As a result of this ruling, the juvenile court now provides detained juveniles with due process. Keep in mind that if Gault had been over eighteen years of age, the maximum punishment would have been a fine up to $50 or imprisonment up to two months. Instead, he received a six-year sentence to a state school without due process. Clearly, the Supreme Court's ruling was critical to the field of children's rights (Hawes, 1991).

Another important case in the area of education was *Pennsylvania Association for Retarded Children (PARC) v. Commonwealth of Pennsylvania* (1972). PARC was a special interest group that advocated for children with intellectual disabilities. The case went to federal court because the state of Pennsylvania denied intellectually impaired children access to public schools. PARC argued that this was unconstitutional. The federal court agreed. The Court ruled that children with intellectual disabilities were entitled to a public education and that their Fourteenth Amendment rights were violated by the state. The case has historical significance because it is seen as the grounding for the passage of the Education of All Handicapped Children Act in 1975.

The rights of children with disabilities were greatly expanded with the passage of the Education of All Handicapped Children Act. Children with disabilities found new rights that they had never known before the passage of this law. The original law is now titled the Individuals with Disabilities Education Act (IDEA). Core provisions of this law include the following:

1. Special needs children are entitled to a free, appropriate education.
2. A child who qualifies for special education services must have an Individual Education Program (IEP). This plan outlines the educational program and services the child is supposed to receive. Recent changes in 1999 under IDEA mandate that parents must have meaningful involvement in placement decisions in special education and the development of the IEP.
3. IDEA requires that parents be given access to all records relating to their special needs child, not just those "relevant" records on the identification, evaluation, and educational placement of their child in special education.

4. IDEA requires that the state have a voluntary mediation process available in case parents disagree with the school district's handling of their child's special education needs. The state is required to pay for the cost of mediation.
5. Parents have a right to a due process hearing if other strategies of mediation do not work. If parents prevail in this hearing, the school district must pay the parents' legal fees and court costs.
6. IDEA requires that parents be informed about the educational progress of their children at least as often as parents of children without disabilities.

Section 504 of the Rehabilitation Act of 1973 and the Americans with Disabilities Act of 1990 (ADA) have also provided important protections for children with disabilities. According to Morrissey (1993), the core principles guiding the ADA in educational settings include the following:

1. The program, service, or activity, when viewed in its entirety, must be readily accessible to and usable by people with disabilities.
2. A person with a disability must be able to access and act on information about a program, service, or activity.
3. When evaluating students with disabilities, screening and testing procedures must be fair, accurate, and nondiscriminatory.
4. Students with disabilities must be able to participate in an activity, service, or program offered to other students.

The philosophical grounding of the ADA was Section 504 of the Rehabilitation Act of 1973. Section 504 and the ADA simply enhance the rights of children with disabilities under IDEA.

Other important cases concerning children's rights were *Doe v. Matava* (Hawes, 1991). This case was filed in Massachusetts on behalf of maltreated children. The case was settled in 1984 when an agreement was reached that Massachusetts had to improve its child welfare system. *Joseph A. v. New Mexico Department of Human Services* was a similar case (Hawes, 1991). The Adoption Assistance and Child Welfare Act of 1980 was the basis for this case (Hawes, 1991). The court ruled that the Adoption Assistance and Child Welfare Act was violated and that state bureaucrats had to follow this national policy with regard to children in the child welfare system. Hawes (1991) concludes that these cases established the following premises concerning children's rights within the child welfare system:

1. Children and citizen's groups now had the right to sue the government.
2. Issues involving children's rights became a federal concern as the result of litigation.
3. Representatives of children could now sue government agencies to challenge the quality of services they provide.
4. Laws such as the Adoption Assistance and Child Welfare Act have created constitutionally protected liberty interests for children.

Attorneys have played a critical role in the area of children's rights. The role of attorneys in helping to ensure that children are entitled to certain rights has created important changes in the juvenile court, public education, and child welfare systems.

IMPORTANT CHILD WELFARE POLICIES AFFECTING CHILDREN'S RIGHTS

The following summarizes important child welfare policies. A number of these policies were mentioned previously in this chapter, others were not. All of these policies affect children's rights because they provide critical protections for children and better define the rights of children in the juvenile justice and child welfare systems (Downs et al., 2004).

Child Abuse Prevention and Treatment Act of 1974 (CAPTA) P.L. 93-247

This policy defines the term child maltreatment. It established a National Center on Child Abuse and Neglect that serves as a clearinghouse for the development and transmittal of information on child protection research and demonstration programs. The policy also provides technical assistance to states and allocates federal funds for child abuse and neglect.

The Indian Child Welfare Act of 1978 (ICWA) P.L. 95-608

Defines the term *Indian child.* This policy mandates that tribes have exclusive jurisdiction over child welfare issues involving an Indian child. It provides specific procedures to ensure compliance by the states.

Adoption and Safe Families Act of 1997 (ASFA) P.L. 105-89 (amended significant provisions of the Adoption Assistance and Child Welfare Act of 1980)

Presents the "reasonable efforts" that must be made by state social service agencies to terminate parental rights. Requires permanency planning hearings within twelve months of out-of-home placement and initiation of a termination of parental rights proceeding when a child has been in care for fifteen of the last twenty-two months, except if the child is with a relative. Reaffirms reasonable efforts and the reunification philosophy expressed under the Adoption Assistance and Child Welfare Act of 1980. The policy promotes timely adoptions through provisions of incentives and funds for postadoption services.

Multiethnic Placement Act of 1994 P.L. 103-382 as amended by the Interethnic Placement Provisions of 1996

This policy prohibits the delay or denial of foster home or adoption placement on the basis of race, color, or national origin of the child or the potential foster or adoptive parent.

Foster Care Independence Act/John H. Chafee Foster Care Independence Program of 1999 (FCLVChafee) P.L. 106-169 (replaced the former Title IV-E Independent Living Program)

Provides flexible funding to states to develop and implement independent living services to remain in foster care until age eighteen. Provides funding for room and board to youth who have left care and are less than twenty-one years old and provides Medicaid coverage of former foster children through twenty-one years.

Juvenile Justice and Delinquency Prevention Act of 1974 (JJDPA) P.L. 93-415 as amended by P.L. 107-273 (2002)

Separates juvenile offenders from adult offenders in detention and places status offenders in secure detention facilities only if they have violated a court order and secure detention is found to be the only way to contain them. Establishes the Office of Juvenile Justice and Delinquency Prevention (OJJDP) and requires compliance as condition for states to receive federal funding for prevention and treatment services.

CHILD ADVOCATES

The *In re Gault* ruling created the need for greater involvement of child advocates to help ensure children have due process in the juvenile justice system. The roles that developed providing this function are guardians ad litem (GAL) and Court Appointed Special Advocates (CASA). The passage of the Child Abuse Prevention and Treatment Act of 1974 made it mandatory to appoint a GAL to represent the best interest of an abused or neglected child in the juvenile justice system. The law did not specify that the GAL had to be an attorney. In 1976, Judge Soukup, then the presiding judge of King County Superior Court in Seattle, Washington, began to look for alternative ways to make sure the best interest of a child would be consistently presented in court. Judge Soukup created the CASA program as a strategy to ensure that the rights of children are protected in the juvenile court and child welfare systems. CASA has grown to include 800 programs nationwide.

CASA volunteers are not trained attorneys. A study by Duquettte and Ramsey (1987) reported that even though CASA volunteers do not have formal legal training, they appear to be as effective as attorneys in the Juvenile Court system. These kinds of findings endorse the importance of lay volunteers to the children's rights movement.

The American Bar Association (ABA) has begun to recognize the need for attorneys to be active in all aspects of the juvenile justice system. Hawes (1991) reports that the ABA and other legal organizations continue to see a number of unmet legal needs of children in the juvenile justice system. These include:

1. The need for clear standards for working with families of children in this system.
2. The need for clear standards for termination of parental rights.
3. The need to create a special children's services division within the juvenile court system that would provide public defenders.
4. The need for clear statutes defining the role of the GAL and CASA volunteer.
5. The need to provide legal counsel for children in custody cases.

Even though lay volunteers can be extremely effective as advocates for the best interests of children, attorneys continue to play the central role in the expansion and clarification of children's rights. Hawes (1991) concludes that attorneys are probably the most effective foot soldiers in the children's rights movement.

Hawes (1991) also argues that child advocates have created a new awareness in all professionals who work with children. Specifically, the children's rights movement has influenced new ethical responsibilities for professionals in the following ways:

1. It has challenged professionals to examine the origins of their beliefs concerning a child's best interest.
2. It has revealed the complexity of protecting children in their routine procedures.
3. It has helped to expose the autocratic use of individual professional's power and judgment in the child welfare and juvenile justice systems.
4. It has stimulated professionals to reconsider ways of responding to parents and children.
5. It has helped to identify the gaps in services, discrepancies between the way children should be served and the way in which they are actually served, and the need to improve policies protecting children.
6. It has underlined the necessity for professionals to go beyond traditional ethical guidelines and to take personal risks to serve children's best interests.

As more professionals join the children's rights movement, they must recognize the importance of the movement to their ethical responsibilities to children, as well as their own beliefs and practices. The following quote from Hawes (1991) succinctly summarizes the importance of the children's rights movement to professionals and the larger society:

> In the 1960s the nation began again to look at the needs of children. At a time when the civil rights movement was in full swing and many middle-class women, the traditional advocates of children's interests, came to see themselves as an oppressed group, the Children's Bureau, the Child Welfare League, social workers, teachers, day-care workers, parents' organizations, and so on, saw the need for organized campaigns if any changes in the way the United States treated its children were to be made. The modern children's rights movement was born, and its members would attract public attention, influence the course of legislation, and, when necessary, file litigation to see that children's rights were acknowledged and enforced. (p. xii)

SUMMARY AND CONCLUSION

As suggested in this chapter, one of the greatest assaults on children's rights, especially for children of low-income families, is not having access to health care and social services. Even though many new rights have emerged for children since the 1960s, poverty continues to be a problem that affects one in four children. Clearly the programs aimed at alleviating poverty are not effective (Piven and Cloward, 1971).

The children's rights movement has been instrumental in the creation of national policies aimed at improving the lives of children in substitute care. Attention must be paid to the psychological reaction of children when placed in foster care and adoption.

The constitutionalization of children's rights has resulted from litigation such as *In re Gault* and *Pennsylvania Association for Retarded Children (PARC) v. Commonwealth of Pennsylvania*. A number of noted authorities such as Goldstein, Freud, and Solnit (1973) influenced the development of national policies that have had a major impact on the rights of children.

This chapter suggests that the welfare reform of 1996 is less than supportive of families. Under HR 3734, TANF and Medicaid are no longer entitlement programs for children and their families. These changes have a negative impact on children's rights. Furthermore, the rules for receiving TANF and Medicaid vary significantly from state to state. For example, this means a child living in Arkansas is treated much differently in terms of economic and medical support than a child in New York.

It was stressed that child advocates have played and will continue to play a critical role in the children's rights movement. Furthermore, advocating for the rights of children is seen as a core responsibility for practitioners working with children.

Chapter 2

The Rights of Parents and Children

According to Westman (1991), under eighteenth century English common law, children were regarded as chattels of their parents and wards of the state—under this system children had no legal rights. Gradually children began to procure legal rights as an outgrowth of the protective doctrine of *parens patriae,* which justifies state intervention into family life under certain circumstances (Westman, 1991). During the twentieth century, the rights of children slowly began to emerge in the United States. The children's rights movement has been largely responsible for the protections now extended to children from the state. The following quote summarizes the current position of children's and parents' rights within the United States (Westman, 1991):

> In practice, the legal adjudication of parent-child rights occurs largely when protection of a child's interests is an issue. The state has the power to intervene and assume temporary custody or guardianship of children when neglect, abuse, or parental incompetence exists. Children can be placed in foster care, and parental rights can be permanently terminated. The state exercises responsibility for determining custody in divorce cases and for establishing a legal parent-child relationship through adoption. Unfortunately, criteria for making these decisions are not well-defined, so that the general practice is to exercise judicial restraint and perpetuate the status quo rather than resolve issues in a timely and definitive manner for a child's benefit. For example, many youngsters spend years in foster care, because no one has assumed the responsibility for making the definitive decisions that are necessary in the legal pursuit of their interests. (p. 47)

What is clear from this quote is that legal rights for children cannot be considered apart from the rights of their parents and the state. Furthermore, the legal criteria for state intervention into family life is not well defined.

DANGERS OF STATE INTERFERENCE

Freeman (1997) argues that state intrusion into family life can make a bad situation even worse. An example of this is well documented in *The Politics of Child Abuse in America* by Costin, Stoesz, and Karger (1997). They argue that the child welfare system in the United States is heavily politicized and does not benefit abused and neglected children or their parents. It is their position that child welfare policy, particularly child abuse policy, contains dangerous contradictions. A rapidly expanding child abuse industry, consisting of enterprising psychotherapists and attorneys, heavily benefits financially from child abuse policy. At the same time, children who are abused and supposed to be protected by the child welfare system are not.

Another problem with state intervention into family life is that the standards that guide this intrusion are not very clear and at times arbitrary. An excellent example of this is the "best interest" standard that has emerged in the field of child welfare. According to Westman (1991) this standard is often based on middle-class values and may at times be seen as a reason for placing children in more affluent or educated families. What this means is that children may be removed from a family because the family is simply poor.

Mnookin (1973) suggests that it is also difficult to determine the "best interest" of a child. Westman (1991) concludes that the child's "best interest" may be fashioned primarily to meet the needs of competing adult claimants or to protect the general policies of agencies. Under these conditions the needs of the child are often secondary.

Freeman (1997) concludes that vague child abuse and neglect laws increase the likelihood that state intervention will be harmful to children. Decisions to remove children from parents under these conditions are often based more on the personal values of authorities than the interest of the child. Freeman (1997) notes that the treatment of children is often based more on cultural biases than rational law. In the area of parental discipline, for example, middle-class parents place a high value on internalized norms of behavior, whereas working-class parents are more prone to use physical punishment. Regional and racial differences as well as class differences exist in the area of child discipline. Given these cultural differences and the vagueness of child abuse and neglect laws, those groups with more power and influence are likely to drive the interpretation of these laws. Clearly the middle-class has the greatest influence in this area. Thus the poor and racial minorities are more likely to have their children removed and placed in substitute care (Costin, Stoesz, and Karger, 1996).

Westman (1991) argues that one strategy that might be used to create more equitable child welfare laws would be the use of the "least detrimental available alternative" standard. Under this standard, realistic available alternatives are considered that bring the least harm to the child. It offers the prospect for a child to maintain a relationship with at least one significant adult, who is or will become the child's psychological parent.

Westman (1991) provides an example of how the "least detrimental" standard works. If one weighs the negatives between abortion and birth control for adolescent children, the "least detrimental" standard of the two can be easily identified. Given the extraordinary social costs of teenage pregnancy, its prevention by contraception can be viewed as the lesser evil. This standard helps to reduce the vagueness surrounding the "best interest" standard through the use of more rational means. It also, for example, provides more privacy and personal choice for adolescent children. Westman (1991) concludes that the challenge for judges and child advocates is to apply the "least detrimental" standard to individual cases with an awareness of their indeterminacy and the long-term impact of current decisions.

Interest in the social and legal rights of children often creates controversy, particularly in relation to the scope of state intervention and the allocation of child-rearing responsibilities between parents and the state. The thrust of child advocacy is aimed at the need to change the discriminatory status of children and make the child's needs primary. At the same time, many in the United States express a strong desire to assure parental autonomy and privacy in child rearing to the fullest extent possible, except in instances where children are clearly and seriously harmed by their parents' child-rearing preferences and practices.

The work of Goldstein, Freud, and Solnit (1973) describes a frame of reference and some procedural prescriptive guidelines for the state to intervene into family life. They attempted to integrate two value preferences: (1) to use the law to make the child's needs paramount and (2) to emphasize privacy in child rearing free of governmental intervention, except in cases of abuse, neglect, and abandonment. They suggest the dangers of state intervention can be tempered by the following strategies.

First, placement decisions should safeguard the child's need for continuity in relationships. The continuity of relationships, including the child's surroundings and environment, are essential for normal child development. Child placements, including custody after divorce and adoption, should stress permanency for the child. Only then can the necessary bonding take place between the child and the psychological parent. The psychological parent is not necessarily the biological parent.

Second, placement decisions should reflect the child's sense of time rather than that of the parents or other adults. Time to a child is dramatically different than what it is for an adult. The child's sense of time affects his or her capacity to cope with breaks in continuity from significant others. The understanding of time through the eyes of a child should be an important factor considered by the court when making placement determinations. The focus of the court should be on children's absence of tolerance to be away from significant adults in their lives.

The third guideline that child placement decisions must take into account is the law's incapacity to supervise interpersonal relationships and the limits of knowledge in making long-range predictions. The state cannot compel a bonding relationship to occur between a child and adult. The court should favor private interpersonal relationships over state-mandated relationships. The court should attempt to identify the psychological parent when placement is needed. If this is not possible, a person should be identified as the potential psychological parent, such as an adoptive parent.

The final guideline is that placement should provide the "least detrimental" standard for safeguarding the child's growth and development. The "best interest" standard, as discussed earlier, is extremely difficult to identify, whereas the "least detrimental" standard emphasizes a rational approach to the court's decision making that emphasizes the needs of the child over other conflicting interests.

JUSTIFYING STATE INTERVENTION

Freeman (1997) argues that a strong case can be made for the state not to intervene into family life. However, by not intervening, the balance between children's and parental rights no longer exist. According to Freeman (1997), the following provides the conditions under which state intervention may be justified.

State intervention can be justified when a parent requests that the court determine the custody of children. For example, when parents separate and they fail to arrive at a custody agreement, the court must make this decision for them.

A second situation would be where familial bonds or psychological parentage exists with a substitute caregiver. These caregivers would include a foster parent or relative who wishes to have legal custody of a child. The other important aspect of this situation is when the biological parent refuses to give up custody. Under these conditions, the court must decide what is best for the child.

A third reason for state intervention is the death or disappearance of both parents, or when parents fail to provide for a child's needs. When parents die or abandon a child, custody decisions can be more easily made; however, they become more clouded when authorities are attempting to decide if parents are meeting the needs of a child.

A fourth reason for state intervention, when parents sexually and physically abuse children, is somewhat more difficult to determine than the others. As covered in Chapter 1, it is very hard to distinguish those families who are abusive from those which are not. Also, if it is determined that a child has been sexually abused, should the child remain in the home? Furthermore, when the state intervenes because of child abuse, authorities must decide if abuse exists or not. Child abuse also takes many forms, including emotional abuse. We lack clear-cut standards for determining child abuse because of cultural biases and other related issues. Regardless of these problems, children have a right to be free of child maltreatment. State intervention into family life is necessary at times in order to protect children. When the state must intervene into family life, it is critical for the rights of children to be protected. However, child advocates must realize that a child's rights can never be fully realized and understood if they are considered apart from the rights of their parents.

MINORITY STATUS OF CHILDREN

The capacity for children and adolescents to act responsibly is connected to their cognitive, intellectual, and social development. As young people move through the life cycle, they develop the capacity to acquire more rights and responsibilities. Steinberg (1991) suggests the transition point for most adolescents to begin to make sound, independent decisions is around age fifteen.

Steinberg (1991) reports that the susceptibility to parental pressure declines steadily through the child's development. As children move through the life cycle, parents have less influence and the peer group takes on added importance to the child. In other words, elementary school students often follow their parents' wishes. Junior high students begin to distance themselves from parents, but do not necessarily have the internal wherewithal to go against the wishes of their peers. Not until high school are youngsters able to develop true behavioral autonomy, which helps them to make their own decisions in face of parental or peer pressures to do otherwise (Steinberg, 1991).

Steinberg (1991) presents a developmental timetable providing insight into when children can take on new rights and responsibilities. Preadolescents (ten years of age or younger) are not capable of responsible independent or sophisticated decision making. Early adolescents (eleven to fourteen years of age) have distanced themselves from parents; however, they do not have the cognitive or emotional skills necessary to handle independence. A great deal of parental and societal protection is critical for children fourteen years of age and under. Older adolescents (fifteen years of age and older) appear to be reasonably competent at making decisions that are sound. It must be noted, however, that these age groupings are relative to the unique differences found among children of all ages.

Steinberg (1991) also stresses that even though adolescents after the age of fifteen years are capable of making sound decisions, they still need to be protected from the larger society. Many parents struggle with two competing views for helping children learn and develop. One stresses the notion that children need to be protected; the other is that children need to be prepared for the realities of adulthood. The "protectionists" view suggests that parents and society should shield children from the realities of adulthood because these realities have the potential to be dangerous, unsettling, or corrupting if children are exposed to them. The "preparationists" position argues that children must learn through experience; this experience will help them to be better prepared for adulthood. Steinberg (1991) concludes that the "preparationists" approach may have negative consequences for children because they are pushed into an adult world before they have the internal capacities to deal with the realities of this world.

The minority legal status of children should be shaped by where the child falls within the developmental life cycle. Unfortunately, laws and legislation that affect children are often shaped by special interest groups such as merchants, ideologues, and parent organizations; these groups may not necessarily represent the interests and needs of children and adolescents (Westman, 1991).

Legislation has a tendency to restrict and reward privileges to children (Westman, 1991). The restrictive approach is grounded in the position that the role of law and legislation is an important means to protect children. The reward strategy provides for greater liberties to young people that are normally age related.

Laws that restrict privileges, such as those that ban drinking alcohol under age twenty-one or prevent the sale of cigarettes or obscene materials to minors, have been upheld by the courts (Westman, 1991). Laws that provide privileges to minors are often related to health issues. For example, the United States Supreme Court in *Planned Parenthood v. Danforth* (1976) found that a blanket rule that requires all minors to get consent from parents to procure an abortion was unconstitutional. Even though the high court made this ruling, the question of whether parents must be notified prior to a minor having an abortion is still unsettled (Westman, 1991). There also continues to be confusion over whether a minor needs parental consent before having access to contraceptives, rehabilitation for substance abuse, and treatment for sexually transmitted disease. Westman, however, makes the following conclusion about the rights of minors: "There is growing statutory recognition that children's interests should be paramount when they conflict with the personal interests of their parents, while safeguarding the legitimate rights of parents to raise their children as they see fit" (p. 53). Keeping this quote in mind, child advocates must realize that children depend on the court system to define their rights as minors. This means the courts are one of the most important mechanisms to ensure the rights of children.

THE LEGAL RIGHTS OF CHILDREN AND PARENTS

It is critical for children to have legal rights in order to protect their interests. The developmental capacity for autonomous decision making, however, is age related. Given this constraint, Westman (1991) outlines the rights of children as follows:

1. Children must have legal rights to protection.
2. Unlimited freedom will stunt children's growth.
3. Children need protection against their own immaturity.
4. Children's rights always include the following
   - Right to food
   - Right to shelter
   - Right to clothing
   - Right to medical care through statutory definition of child abuse
   - Right to be protected from the harmful acts of others
   - Certain rights are age-graded, for example, obtaining a driver's license and voting eligibility.

As the child moves through the life cycle, additional rights can be granted. Westman warns, however, that the adolescent must be allowed to test his or her capacity for responsibility. If he or she is not given this opportunity to do so, maturation is delayed and rebellion may well be the outcome.

Parents' rights at times conflict with the rights of children. An example of this is the case of *Wisconsin v. Yoder* (1972). The United States ruled in this case that Amish parents could remove their children from public school at age fourteen. One could argue that the rights of the child have been violated in this case. The rights of the child typically prevail over the rights of parents in health-related issues, such as in *Planned Parenthood v. Danforth*.

Westman (1991) suggests the following are core rights of parents. Parents have the right:

1. To name children
2. To custody of children
3. To control a child's religion and education
4. To discipline children
5. To decide where a child lives
6. To decide what children will eat
7. To decide how children will dress
8. To censor the books read, video games played, and movies seen by children.

Children's rights are least protected in the privacy of the home. Westman also argues that the state should be reluctant to intervene into family life for a number of reasons. First, state intervention undermines the attractiveness of parenthood. Second, parenthood is a sacrificial burden; state intervention makes this burden even less attractive. Last, state intervention may undermine parental authority.

CHILD LIBERATIONISTS VERSUS CHILD PROTECTIONISTS

Few would deny the importance of children having rights that help to ensure they are protected from the dangers of the larger society. Rights allow people to stand with dignity and, if necessary, to demand their due without having to grovel, please, or beg. If one has rights one is entitled to respect and dignity—no amount of benevolence or compassion can be an adequate substitute (Freeman, 1997).

The children's rights movement is largely a product of the twentieth century. Two schools of thought have driven the philosophical grounding of the children's rights movement. One approach, child liberation, suggests that children are entitled to self-determination; the other, child protection, argues that children need to be nurtured and protected by society.

Those advocating for allowing children to have self-determination fall under what has been coined the children's liberation movement. This movement has been influenced by Farson's (1974) work titled

Birthrights. Holt, in his book *Escape from Childhood* (1974), developed core positions underpinning the children's liberation movement.

Farson (1974) argued that self-determination is the root of all rights that children are entitled to claim. Farson anticipated the criticism to his position with the following argument:

> We will grant children rights for the same reason we grant rights to adults, not because we are sure that children will then become better people, but more for ideological reasons, because we believe that expanding freedom as a way of life is worthwhile in itself. And freedom, we have found, is a difficult burden for adults as well as for children. (p. 31)

Farson identified a number of rights based on self-determination that he felt children should be entitled to:

1. The right to alternative home environments—allowing the child to choose his or her living arrangements;
2. The right to information that is accessible to adults, such as being allowed to inspect records kept about them;
3. The right to educate oneself and to abolish compulsory education;
4. The right to sexual freedom;
5. The right to economic power, including the right to work and to develop a credit record and to achieve economic independence;
6. The right to political power, including the right to vote;
7. The right to freedom from abuse and neglect; and
8. The right to justice and fair treatment in the courts.

Holt (1974) proposed the following eleven rights that children should be granted:

1. The right to equal treatment at the hands of the law;
2. The right to vote and to take part in the political system;
3. The right to be legally responsible for one's acts;
4. The right to work;
5. The right to privacy in one's home;
6. The right to financial independence and responsibility;
7. The right to choose one's own education;

8. The right to travel and to live away from home;
9. The right to receive from the state the same income supports received by adults;
10. The right to make and enter into quasifamilial relationships outside one's immediate family; and
11. The right to do what adults are allowed to do.

As would be suspected, the greatest resistance to children's liberation comes from parents, teachers, and children themselves (Hawes, 1991). Parents and teachers are heavily grounded in the child protectionists' view. Child advocates who push various agendas designed to improve conditions for children in society as a whole, in the schools, in families, and in the juvenile justice system also fall under the protectionists' philosophy (Hawes, 1991).

Child protectionists are advocates for children's rights; however, they are not willing to grant full autonomy or adulthood to minors. They define children's rights in terms of claims on the larger society, whereas child liberationists believe that the granting of complete legal freedom will enable children to protect themselves (Hawes, 1991).

Several issues have arisen from the debate between child liberationists and protectionists. They differ most dramatically on the role of adults in improving conditions of children in society (Hawes, 1991). Child liberationists argue there would be little or no need for adults to intervene on behalf of children if they were given full legal rights (Farson, 1974). In contrast, child protectionists argue that they must continue to work toward improving the rights of children and to ensure that children receive protections from the dangers of the larger society (Hawes, 1991).

U.S. SUPREME COURT RULINGS DEFINING THE RIGHTS OF PARENTS AND CHILDREN

The decisions and reasoning of the Supreme Court in the area of parent and child rights and interests is complex and at first appear to be contradictory. With careful review and analysis, however, the decisions become more cogent and clear. A core reason for the variance is that Supreme Court decisions interpret public policy matters that often create conflicting needs and goals of parents, children, and society. The cases that are reviewed in this section are weighted in the direction of reinforcing the rights of parents in the upbringing of their children. Some limit the rights of parents. Others extend and limit the legal rights of minors (Downs et al., 2004).

Decisions Reinforcing Parental Rights

The primary rights and responsibilities of caring for children rest with their parents. These rights and responsibilities were outlined earlier in the chapter. The following cases focus on Supreme Court rulings that reinforce the rights of parents (Kramer, 2004).

Pierce v. Society of Sisters, *1925*

The state of Oregon required parents of children between the ages of eight and sixteen years to send their children to public schools. A number of private schools brought action on behalf of themselves and the parents of children attending their schools, claiming the law was unconstitutional. The Supreme Court ruled that a state could not require parents to send their children to only public schools.

Wisconsin v. Yoder, *1972*

The state of Wisconsin required parents to send their children to either public or private school until the age of sixteen years. Amish parents refused to send their fourteen- and fifteen-year-old children to school after completion of the eighth grade because of religious beliefs. The Court concluded that accommodating the religious objections of the Amish by forgoing one, or at most two, additional years of compulsory education would not impair the physical and mental health of the child, or result in an inability to be self-supporting or to discharge the duties and responsibilities of citizenship, or in any other way materially detract from the welfare of society. Thus the Court ruled in favor of the parents.

Palmore v. Sidoti, *1984*

This Florida child-custody case involved a white couple who divorced when their child was three years old. Custody was granted to the mother, who subsequently married an African American. The father petitioned for custody of the child and a Florida court awarded him custody. The case was appealed to the Supreme Court. The Court ruled in favor of the mother and argued that even though the reality of private biases and the possible injury they might inflict are permissible considerations for removal of an infant child from the custody of its natural mother, the Constitution cannot control such prejudices but neither can it tolerate them.

Parliam v. J. R., *1979*

A Supreme Court decision was made in this case challenging the rights of parents to institutionalize their children for mental health treatment and of the state to institutionalize its wards (that is, children under its supervision and/or in its custody) without due process procedures. The neglected child in this case was removed from his natural parents at three months and placed in several different foster homes prior to admission to the state hospital at seven years of age on request of the Georgia Department of Family and Children Services. The child was assessed to be borderline retarded with an unsocialized, aggressive reaction of childhood. On these facts, the Court ruled that the traditional presumption that natural bonds of affection lead parents to act in the best interests of their children should apply. Parents should retain a substantial if not the dominant role in the decision to voluntarily commit their children to an institution. Furthermore, Georgia law provided for informal medical review thirty days after admission to state hospitals, and the Court underscored as protection to the child the authority of doctors to make medical judgments. Thus the decision reinforced not only the authority of parents and agents of the state over children, but also the authority of the medical profession in confining children for medical intervention (Downs et al., 2004).

Santosky v. Kramer, *1982*

The New York law provided that a child could be declared permanently neglected using a "fair preponderance of the evidence" standard, and on this basis the court could permanently terminate parental rights. The Santoskys lost custody of three children on petitions filed by the local Department of Social Services alleging neglect of the oldest child, physical abuse of the second child, and "immediate removal necessary to avoid imminent danger to his life or health" of the third child within three days of birth. The children were placed in foster care for five years before a petition to terminate parental rights was filed (Downs et al., 2004).

While the Santosky children were in foster care the parents were provided a number of services to improve their parenting skills. The Department of Social Services concluded that the parents did not take advantage of the services offered and their parental rights were terminated. The parents appealed, alleging that the New York statute under which the termination of their rights occurred violated the due process clause of the Fourteenth Amendment. The Court concluded that the parent's due process rights were violated (Downs et al., 2004).

Troxel v. Granville, *2000*

This case focused on third-party visitation rights over the objection of the parent. The Troxels were paternal grandparents to two children, whose mother was Granville. Granville and the children's father, who were not married, ended their relationship in 1991. The father lived with his parents, the Troxels, until he committed suicide in 1993. During the time he resided with his parents, the children visited in the Troxel's home on a weekly basis. After the death of father, the Troxels continued to see the children regularly. In October 1993, Granville told them she wished to limit their visitation to one visit per month. The Troxels filed a court petition in December 1993 requesting two weekends of overnight visitation per month and two weeks of visitation each summer (Downs et al., 2004). The state of Washington's statute at Section 26.10.160(3) states, "any person may petition for visitation rights at any time including, but not limited to, custody proceedings. The court may grant such visitation rights whenever visitation may serve the best interests of the child whether or not there has been any change of circumstances." Granville did not oppose all visitation. However, she asked the court to limit the visitation to one day per month. The Washington Superior Court entered an order in 1995 granting visitation one weekend per month, one week during the summer, and four hours on both of the petitioning grandparents' birthdays (Downs et al., 2004).

Granville appealed to the Washington Court of Appeals; since there were no written findings of facts and conclusions of law, the Washington Court of Appeals remanded the case to the Superior Court. The Superior Court, in its written opinion, found that visitation was in the children's best interests. However, when the case was appealed to the Washington Supreme Court, this court concluded that the rights of natural parents would be potentially violated by allowing visitations when parents objected to these visits. The case was ultimately appealed to the United States Supreme Court, which concluded that parents had the fundamental right to make decisions concerning the care, custody, and control of their children. Thus parents had the right to control visitations; this means, for example, that parents can deny visitation by grandparents if a child has been placed in foster care or some other related family setting.

Ferguson v. City of Charleston, *2001*

This case focuses on the constitutionality of a policy developed by a Charleston public hospital, in cooperation with law enforcement. This policy provided that the hospital would order urine drug screens on women suspected of using cocaine, report women who tested positive for cocaine to the local police, and refer them for substance abuse treatment. The record is not clear as to the specificity of consent to testing for drug use required by the women (Downs et al., 2004).

Ten women who received obstetrical care at the hospital were ultimately arrested. The women challenged the validity of the policy. The Supreme Court ultimately found the policy to be unconstitutional on the grounds that there is a reasonable expectation of privacy enjoyed by the typical patient undergoing diagnostic tests in a hospital and that the results of those tests would not be shared with non-medical personnel without patient consent (Downs et al., 2004).

In summary, the Supreme Court decisions have established that parents have a right to choose to send their children to a public or a private school; to refuse to adhere to compulsory school attendance statutes when they conflict with religious beliefs; to institutionalize their children for treatment provided there are appropriate assessment and periodic reviews that support the need for the institutionalization;

to have a clear standard of proof applied in proceedings to terminate their rights; to have their decisions about third-party visitations with their children given weight in court proceedings; and to be free from nonconsensual drug screenings during pregnancy (Downs et al., 2004).

Decisions Limiting Parental Rights

The Supreme Court has also issued decisions that have limited parental rights. The following is a summary of those cases.

Prince v. Massachusetts, *1944*

In this case, Massachusetts enacted a law that prohibited children under twelve years of age from selling newspapers, magazines, and periodicals in public places. Furthermore, it was unlawful for parents or guardians to permit a minor to engage in such behavior. The aunt of a nine-year-old girl gave her Jehovah's Witness magazines, *Watchtower* and *Consolation,* to distribute on the streets at 5 cents per copy. The aunt was convicted of violating the Massachusetts' law. Her case was appealed ultimately to the U.S. Supreme Court alleging that the Massachusetts law violated her free exercise of religion provision in the First Amendment. The Supreme Court concluded that parents may be free to become martyrs themselves, but it does not follow that they are free, in identical circumstances, to make martyrs of their children before they have reached the age of full and legal discretion, when they can make that choice for themselves (Downs et al., 2004).

Baltimore City Department of Social Services v. Rouknight, *1990*

Rouknight was the mother of an adjudicated abused child, Maurice, who was in her custody under the supervision of Baltimore City Department of Social Services (BCDSS). A petition was filed to return the child to foster care because of the mother's failure to follow the court-ordered treatment plan. Rouknight refused to produce the child; she was held in contempt and imprisoned until she produced the child or revealed to the court his whereabouts. She appealed, claiming the order violated her Fifth Amendment rights. The Court of Appeals of Maryland found the contempt order unconstitutional; however, when the case was appealed to the Supreme Court, the Court reversed the judgment of the Maryland Court of Appeals. The Court argued that once the child was adjudicated and in need of assistance, his care and safety became the particular object of the state's regulatory interests. Furthermore, when accepting care of Maurice subject to the custodial order's conditions, Rouknight submitted to the routine operation of the regulators' system and agreed to hold Maurice in a manner consonant with the state's regulatory interests and subject to inspection by BCDSS (Downs et al., 2004).

In sum, the Supreme Court has supported the states by allowing them greater authority than parents in the regulation and enforcement of child labor and child protection.

Reproductive Rights of Minors

The following cases focus on the rights of minors to control their own reproductive capacities by access to contraception or abortion.

Roe v. Wade, *1973*

In this case the Supreme Court granted a constitutional protection allowing women the right to choose abortion early in pregnancy and the right of the state to regulate the termination of pregnancy after viability of the fetus, that is, when the life of the unborn child may be continued indefinitely outside the womb by natural or artificial life-supportive systems (Downs et al., 2004).

Planned Parenthood v. Danforth, *1976*

In this Missouri case, the state required the written consent of a parent or person in loco parentis for an abortion during the first twelve weeks of pregnancy of an unmarried woman under the age of eighteen years unless there was a certification by a physician that abortion was necessary to preserve the life of the minor. The Supreme Court found that the Missouri law was unconstitutional and concluded that the state may not impose a blanket provision requiring the consent of a parent or person in loco parentis as a condition for abortion of an unmarried minor during the first twelve weeks of her pregnancy. Just as with the requirement of consent from the spouse, so here, the state does not have the constitutional authority to give a third party an absolute, and possibly arbitrary, veto over the decision of the physician and his or her patient to terminate the patient's pregnancy, regardless of the reason for withholding the consent (Downs et al., 2004).

Bellotti v. Baird, *1979*

In this case, a Massachusetts law required a pregnant unmarried minor to have the consent of her parent or the permission of a judge before she could obtain an abortion. Massachusetts passed this law after the *Danforth* decision and provided an alternative procedure that required the permission of a judge to ensure that the parents did not have absolute veto authority over whether their minor should receive an abortion. The Supreme Court concluded that although the law satisfied constitutional standards in large part, it fell short in two respects: First, it permited judicial authorization for an abortion to be withheld from a minor who is mature and fully competent to make this decision independently. Second, it required parental notification in every instance, without affording the pregnant minor an opportunity to receive an independent judicial determination that she is mature enough to consent or that an abortion would be in her best interests (Downs et al., 2004).

H. L. v. Matheson, *1981*

In this case, a Utah law required a physician to notify, if possible, the parents or guardians of a minor on whom the physician intended to perform an abortion. Neither the parents nor judges had veto power over the minor's abortion decision. A physician had advised a fifteen-year-old pregnant girl, living with her parents, that an abortion would be in the minor's best medical interests. Because of the criminal liability involved, he refused to perform the abortion without notifying the minor's parents. The girl argued that this notification requirement restricted her right to privacy and violated the doctor-patient relationship. The Supreme Court upheld the law and argued that the fact that the requirement of parental notice may inhibit some minors from seeking abortions is not a valid basis to void the law. In other words, the law plainly serves important state interests, is narrowly drawn to protect only those interests, and does not violate any guarantees of the Constitution (Downs et al., 2004).

Ohio v. Akron Center for Reproductive Health, *1990*

An Ohio law required a physician or other person contemplating performing an abortion on a pregnant unmarried person under the age of eighteen to notify at least one parent or to have a judge's order permitting the abortion. To secure an abortion, a judge must have clear and convincing proof that that the minor has sufficient maturity and information to make the abortion decision herself, that one of her parents has engaged in a pattern of maltreatment against her, or that notice is not in her best interests. The Court concluded that it would deny all dignity to the family to say that the state cannot take this reasonable step in regulating its health professions to ensure that, in most cases, a young woman will receive guidance and understanding from a parent (Downs et al., 2004).

Hodgson v. Minnesota, *1990*

In this case, the Supreme Court held unconstitutional the section of Minnesota law requiring physicians or their agents to notify both parents of an unmarried person under the age of eighteen years of the intent to perform an abortion and to wait forty-eight hours before carrying out the procedure; however, the Court held constitutional the section of the law that provided for judicial bypass to two-parent notification when the minor could establish that she was mature and capable of giving informed consent, that she was the victim of parental maltreatment, or that it was in her best interests to have an abortion without notice to one or both of her parents and the judge granted permission to the physician to perform the abortion (Downs et al., 2004).

Carey v. Population Services International, *1977*

A New York law prohibited the sale and distribution of nonprescription contraceptives to minors under the age of sixteen years. The Court found the New York law unconstitutional and concluded that the right to privacy in connection with decisions affecting procreation extends to minors as well as to adults and that inhibiting minors' privacy rights was valid only to serve a significant state interest (Downs et al., 2004).

The Supreme Court has established the following concerning parental authority and the reproductive rights of minors.

- Minors have the right to receive contraceptive services without parental permission.
- Minors have a right to abortions.
- Parents or persons acting in loco parentis do not have absolute veto power over a minor's decision to have an abortion.
- Minors have a right to an independent judicial determination that they are mature enough to make a decision to have an abortion or that the abortion is in the minor's best interests.

However, states may enact laws requiring or permitting notification to a parent of the minor's decision to have an abortion by a medical professional who will perform the abortion (Downs et al., 2004).

Constitutional Rights of Children

The following cases focus on children's rights and responsibilities. These cases largely focus on issues related to the juvenile court system.

Kent v. United States, *1966*

A District of Columbia law provided that a person sixteen years of age or older charged with an offense that would be a felony if committed by an adult could be waived to the adult court for trial. A minor named Kent was charged with robbery, rape, and breaking and entering. His case was waived. Kent challenged the waiver on the grounds that he was not afforded a hearing, no reasons for the waiver were provided to him, and his lawyer was denied access to his records. The Supreme Court concluded that under the due process clause, a juvenile was entitled to a hearing, full access to records and reports used by the court in arriving at the court's decision, and a statement explaining the juvenile court's actions (Downs et al., 2004).

In re Gault, *1967*

Gault, a fifteen-year-old boy, was charged with making a lewd telephone call to a neighbor. He was on probation at the time the call was made and was arrested without notification to his parents, detained, not provided access to an attorney, and not given a formal hearing. Gault was found delinquent and committed to the state training school until the age of majority. The Supreme Court reversed the decision of the Arizona Supreme Court and established the due process requirements for juvenile delinquency hearings, notice of sufficient detail to mount a defense, right to be represented by counsel, privilege against self-incrimination, and the right to review evidence and cross-examine witnesses (Downs et al., 2004).

In re Winship, *1970*

Winship, a twelve-year-old boy, was charged with stealing. He was adjudicated delinquent and the Supreme Court held that the standard of proof in a delinquency case is "beyond a reasonable doubt," the same standard required in adult court (Downs et al., 2004).

McKeiver v. Pennsylvania, *1971*

McKeiver, a sixteen-year-old boy charged with robbery, larceny, and receiving stolen property, was denied a jury trial, adjudicated, and ultimately placed on probation. His attorney challenged the denial of a jury trial. The Court held that the fundamental fairness standard in fact-finding procedures for juvenile proceedings as developed by *Gault* and *Winship* did not require a jury trial. This ruling was a clear indication that the Court wanted to maintain some of the informalities of the juvenile court system (Downs et al., 2004).

Breed v. Jones, *1975*

Jones was a seventeen-year-old male charged with armed robbery. The juvenile court found that he had committed the crime and ultimately determined that he was not suitable for treatment in the juvenile system. He was turned over for prosecution in the adult system. Jones appealed with the claim that this was a violation of the double jeopardy clause of the Fifth Amendment and due process and equal protection as found in the Fourteenth Amendment. The case went to the Supreme Court, which focused on whether Jones could be prosecuted as an adult and if his Fifth and Fourteenth Amendments rights had been violated. The Court ruled that a transfer to adult court for prosecution after an adjudication of delinquency in the juvenile court violates the Fifth Amendment protection against double jeopardy (Downs et al., 2004).

Fare v. Michael C., *1979*

Michael, a sixteen-year-old, was charged with murder. He was taken into custody and advised of his rights under *Miranda*. When he asked to see his probation officer, his request was denied. He provided information about his crime. However, when he was charged with the murder, he sought to have the information he provided to police suppressed because it had been obtained in violation of his *Miranda* rights, as he had been denied access to his probation officer. The Court held that a juvenile's request to speak with his probation officer does not constitute a per se request to remain silent nor is it tantamount to a request for an attorney, because the probation officer does not fulfill the important role in protecting the rights of the accused juvenile that an attorney plays (Downs et al., 2004).

Eddings v. Oklahoma, *1982*

Eddings, a sixteen-year-old boy tried as an adult for first-degree murder of a police officer, was convicted and sentenced to death. Oklahoma law allowed for presentation of evidence of "mitigating circumstances." Eddings offered that he had a history of maltreatment by his father. The judge refused to consider this evidence. The Supreme Court vacated the death sentence and held that the Eighth and Fourteenth Amendments required individualized consideration of mitigating circumstances in capital cases (Downs et al., 2004).

Schall v. Martin, *1984*

This New York law authorized pretrial detention of an accused juvenile delinquent on a finding that there is a serious risk that the minor might commit another offense if not detained pending trial. Martin, a fourteen-year-old boy, was arrested for first-degree robbery, second-degree assault, and criminal possession of a weapon. Martin was detained after lying about where he lived. A hearing was held the following day on a delinquency petition, and he was detained pending trial. After the hearing Martin was adjudicated delinquent and placed on two years' probation. Martin challenged the New York law as violating the due process and equal protection clauses of the Fourteenth Amendment. The Supreme Court held that the referenced statute was not invalid under the due process clause of the Fourteenth Amendment given the regulatory purpose for the detention and the procedural protections that precede its imposition (Downs et al., 2004).

Thompson v. Oklahoma, *1988*

This Oklahoma law provided that juveniles charged with serious offenses could be tried and thus sentenced as adults. Thompson was a fifteen-year-old boy charged with murder who was tried as an adult, convicted, and sentenced to death. The question addressed by the Supreme Court was whether the execution of that sentence would violate the constitutional prohibition against the infliction of cruel and unusual punishment because the petitioner was only fifteen years old at the time of the offense. The Court held that the youth of the defendant—more specifically, the fact that he was less than sixteen years old at the time of his offense—is sufficient reason for denying the state the power to sentence him to death, stating that it is a violation of contemporary standards of decency and that such a young person is not capable of acting with the degree of culpability that can justify the ultimate penalty (Downs et al., 2004).

Stanford v. Kentucky, *1989, and* Wilkins v. Missouri, *1989*

Stanford, a seventeen-year-old boy, committed a murder in Kentucky. The juvenile court transferred the minor for trial as an adult under Kentucky law—he was convicted and sentenced to death. Wilkins was sixteen years old when he committed murder in Missouri—he was also tried as an adult and sentenced to death. The issue before the Supreme Court in both cases was whether the death sentence for a sixteen- or seventeen-year-old constituted cruel and unusual punishment under the Eighth Amendment. The Court ruled that such a punishment does not offend the Eighth Amendment's prohibition against cruel and unusual punishment (Downs et al., 2004).

In summary, for juveniles charged with delinquent/criminal crimes, the Supreme Court has established that juveniles must be afforded due process rights, that states can maintain some flexibility and informality in their juvenile court processes to ensure the benevolent treatment of juveniles, and that juveniles can be sentenced to death (Downs et al., 2004).

Rights of Government

Recognition of the government's role in intervening in the autonomy of the family clearly emerged over the past several decades. The role of government is being further defined and limited by the various decisions by the Supreme Court.

The government's interest in protecting children from harm and protecting society from the delinquent acts of children is rooted in the principle of *parens patriae*. This principle was discussed earlier in this chapter. According to Downs and colleagues (2004), this principle allows government to do the following:

1. If the parents are unwed, state laws are invoked to establish paternity.
2. If the parents separate or divorce, state child custody laws are invoked to determine custody, parenting time (visitation), and support.
3. If the parents are temporarily unable to care for the child, state guardianship laws are invoked to provide for voluntary transfer of guardianship or state child abuse and neglect or juvenile delinquency laws are invoked to provide for court wardship due to dependency, abuse, neglect, or delinquency (involuntary action).
4. If parents are found to be unable or unwilling to remedy the situation that necessitated involuntary action, then state termination of parental rights under child emancipation laws are invoked to permanently terminate their rights and responsibilities (emancipation or termination of parental rights).

5. If new parents are found, state adoption laws are invoked to legally establish a new parenting relationship with all the rights, privileges, and duties afforded biological parents.

SUMMARY AND CONCLUSION

This chapter attempts to present the rights of children and parents in modern American society. The early basis for these rights is grounded in eighteenth century English common law. The doctrine of *parens patriae* emerged from the English legal system. This tradition means the state can intervene into family life when parents do not protect their children from harm. The tension between children's and parent's rights is partially grounded in the doctrine of *parens patriae*.

The dangers of state intervention into family life are presented. However, it is suggested that if the needs of children are protected and the privacy of reasonable child-rearing practices free from government intervention are considered, many of the problems related to state intervention into the affairs of the family can be tempered. If anything, the chapter argues for strong laws and legislation to protect children from harm in their families and the larger society. Many of these cases were reviewed in this chapter.

The debate between the child liberationists and protectionists cannot be easily resolved. The research on child development appears to negate the arguments for child liberation; specifically, as the child protectionists would agree, children do not have the cognitive, intellectual, and emotional development necessary to make sound choices concerning their lives.

Child advocates continue to push for greater protections of children in families and other social systems. As these advocacy efforts result in new laws and legislation, the tension between the rights of children and parents will increase. Westman (1991) summarizes this tension as follows:

> The legal rights of minors cluster around rights to nurturance, protection, and to make autonomous choices. There is a developmental gradient in minors' capacities to perceive, to understand, and to express their views of life circumstances. The

authority of their parents generally is honored because of the presumption that it is based upon love and wisdom. It is based also upon the awareness that parenthood involves sacrificial duties that, in turn, require the cooperation and obedience of children. Theoretically, the interests of parents and children are congruent when an adult is functioning competently in the parenting role. When conflicts arise between the rights of parents and children, they usually are based upon the personal interests of a person outside of the parenting role. (p. 62)

Chapter 3

The Rights of Able Children
and Children with Disabilities in Schools

The children's rights movement within the United States has been driven by the protections granted under the Bill of Rights, the first ten amendments to the Constitution, which guard against unjust and unreasonable actions by government.

Most child advocates agree, however, that children do not have the cognitive and intellectual development to be granted the same rights as adults (Westman, 1991). This premise has guided the development of children's rights in the courts, the child welfare system, and schools. The focus of this chapter is to present the rights of children in schools.

The rights of children in public and private schools have expanded over the past several decades; this is particularly true for children with disabilities. With the passage of the Education of All Handicapped Children Act in 1975, now titled the Individuals with Disabilities Education Act (IDEA), children with disabilities found new rights that they had never known before. General provisions of IDEA include the following:

1. Children with disabilities are entitled to a free, appropriate education.
2. A child who qualifies for special education services must have an individual education program (IEP) that outlines the child's educational program and services he or she will receive.
3. IDEA requires that parents be given access to all records relating to their special needs child.
4. IDEA requires that the state must have a voluntary mediation process if parents disagree with the school district's handling of their child's special education needs.

5. Parents have a right to a due process hearing if other strategies of mediation do not work.
6. IDEA requires that parents be informed about the educational progress of their children at least as often as parents of children without disabilities.

Section 504 of the Rehabilitation Act of 1973 and the Americans with Disabilities Act (ADA) of 1990 have also provided important protections for children with disabilities. The philosophical grounding of the ADA is Section 504 of the Rehabilitation Act of 1973. Section 504 and the ADA simply enhance the rights of children with disabilities under IDEA. What is particularly important about the ADA is that both public and private schools are covered by this law. Private schools that receive federal funding must also meet the requirements of Section 504 of the Rehabilitation Act; these are very similar to the ADA requirements for private schools. Only public schools, however, must meet the legal requirements of IDEA.

This chapter will present the rights of all children in public schools. The focus will then move to the rights of children with disabilities in public and private school settings.

THE RIGHTS OF CHILDREN IN PUBLIC SCHOOLS

The U.S. court system has made important rulings affecting student rights in the public school system. These rulings dealt with issues related to freedom of expression and speech, censorship, and school safety versus privacy. The children's rights movement, through court actions and other advocacy strategies, has helped to ensure that children do not leave their constitutional rights at the public school door.

Freedom of Expression and Speech

The First Amendment grants basic protections to American citizens that allow them to freely express themselves. These include the right to state one's opinions and beliefs, the right to write freely without censorship, and the right to read what they please; however, within the public school, these rights are greatly curtailed (Malaspina, 1998).

When the rights of others in the school system are abused, school officials can limit freedom of expression. For example, in 1995 a group of seniors in a Greenwich, Connecticut, high school secretly placed a racial slur in a yearbook. The students were identified and were not allowed to graduate because of this action. In other words, the First Amendment does not protect messages of bigotry of one student group against another group (Malaspina, 1998).

The freedom of expression through clothing can also be limited by public schools. Limiting freedom of expression is often done on the premise that certain kinds of self-expression may disrupt the education process. For example, in 1996 in Burlington, Vermont, a gay high school student was sent home because he continually wore a dress to school. The school appeared to be within its legal rights by ordering the child home because of his behavior. Another example is the case in Hadley, Massachusetts, where a student was not allowed to wear a T-shirt that a teacher felt was obscene. The local school board upheld the teacher's position and implemented an even stricter dress code (Malaspina, 1998).

Dress codes are perceived by school officials as a deterrent to gang activities that may lead to school violence inside and outside the school. Typically, dress codes prohibit clothing that demeans others on the basis of religion, sex, or race. These kinds of prohibitions appear legal. Malaspina points out, however, that dress codes that simply reflect the taste of policymakers, such as deeming a tie-dyed T-shirt as inappropriate or girls not being allowed to wear pants, can be successfully challenged in the courts by students and their parents.

Censorship

Student written materials can also be curtailed by public schools. In an important court ruling in the 1980s, *Hazelwood School District v. Kuhlmeir* (Malaspina, 1998), the Supreme Court held that educators did not violate the First Amendment rights of students by exercising editorial control over the content and style of student speech in school-sponsored expression activities as long as these actions are reasonable and based on legitimate pedagogical concerns. At issue in the Hazelwood case were the actions of a principal who censored discussion of sexual activity, divorce, and birth control in a student newspaper. This important ruling suggests that public schools can monitor and censor the expression of students in the public school system (Malaspina, 1998). However, this right of the school is not absolute, as suggested under the 1969 Supreme Court ruling of *Tinker v. Des Moines Independent Community School District* (Malaspina, 1998). The justices ruled that students had a right to wear black armbands to school to protest the Vietnam War. Thus, students do not shed all of their rights to freedom of speech or expression when they enter the school (Westman, 1991).

School Safety versus Privacy

Clearly, violence in American schools is an important social problem, as perceived by the public. Recent "zero tolerance" policies in schools have greatly curtailed the privacy rights of students. Public schools have implemented programs aimed at school safety that include the use of metal detectors, random searches of student lockers, and the use of drug-sniffing dogs. Many students are now required to wear identification bands (Malaspina, 1998).

All Americans have a right to privacy under the Fourth Amendment; court rulings, however, suggest that public schools can greatly limit this right. Two notable U.S. Supreme Court rulings, *New Jersey v. T. L. O.* (1985) and *Vernonia School District 47J v. Acton* (1995), support this position (Malaspina, 1998).

New Jersey v. T. L. O. offers a classic case that provides schools with direction on student privacy issues. In this case, the Supreme Court ruled that school searches are constitutional as long as there is reasonable grounds for suspecting that the search will turn up evidence that a student has violated a law or the rules of a school (Malaspina, 1998).

In *Vernonia School District 47J v. Acton,* the Supreme Court allowed for greater latitude in the area of student searches. The Court ruled that the state's interest in attacking the problem of drugs in schools outweighs the student's right to individualized suspicion. This ruling now allows, for example, schools to require drug testing of all students who wish to play sports. Numerous schools presently require random drug testing of athletes and other students. Clearly, the safety of all students in public schools is viewed as more important than a student's right to privacy. However, students do have limited rights of privacy because there generally must be "probable cause" before school officials or police conduct a search on school grounds (Malaspina, 1998).

Student Rights versus School Violence

A recent article by Donohue (1999) suggests that school violence in America is more media hype than reality. She argues that policy-makers, including school boards, are reacting to public opinion, which is largely driven by news outlets that often described school violence as a rising trend in the 1990s. Donohue (1999) presents the following data supporting here position:

1. School-associated violent deaths reveal that children face approximately a one-in-a-million chance of being killed at school. A child has a much higher probability of being struck by lightning.
2. Research generally concludes that since 1972, school shootings have declined.
3. Ninety-nine percent of violence aimed at children occurs outside of school grounds.
4. Research has found that the vast majority of principals report no violence in their schools. Violence is defined as violent crime by murder, suicide, rape, physical attacks, or sexual battery.
5. Less than 1 percent of students between ages twelve and nineteen report being victims of violence in schools.
6. Urban schools are more likely to report serious violent crime; little evidence suggests violent crime is increasing in suburban or rural schools.
7. Eighty-nine percent of urban students and 90 percent of rural students feel safe at school.
8. Most violent crime aimed at children occurs four hours after the ending of school.

These findings provide important insight into the school violence phenomena. These data strongly suggest that much of the school violence problem may well be media hype. Furthermore, in a certain sense, myth is driving the development of public policy aimed at curtailing a problem that may well not exist. Given the fact that many rights of children are already limited by public school systems, further curtailment of these rights because of school violence does not appear warranted.

A number of recent public policy initiatives have been linked to the perception of rising school violence (Donohue, 1999). Some of these policies not only infringe upon the well-being of students but also their rights. These include:

1. The ending of after-school programs. Most authorities agree that after-school programs are one of the most important strategies for creating a safe environment for children after school.
2. President Clinton requested that more police officers be placed in schools, even though 99 percent of juvenile homicides are committed outside of schools.
3. Zero-tolerance policies have resulted in school expulsions and suspensions that are excessive. Children, for example, have been expelled from school for making fake threats aimed at "the Spice Girls" and the television character "Barney," the purple dinosaur.
4. An increasing number of children are being tried as adults. The evidence is very clear that children who are imprisoned with adults are at tremendous risk for sexual abuse and higher rates of recidivism.

Donohue (1999) summarizes the current conflict between student rights and the perceived threat of rising school violence:

> Major criminal justice reform being proposed to remedy the "crisis" of school shootings could fundamentally change the nature of children's rights. While executing the 11-year-old suspect in a school shooting may fit someone's sense of vengeance, it will have dubious, if any, crime-control impact. In reality, homicides committed by children under age 13 occur less frequently today than in 1965. According to the FBI's Uniform Crime Reports, there were 25 homicides by juveniles under 13 in 1965, compared to 16 in 1996—a 36 percent decline. The real threats facing our children won't be dealt with by putting them in jail, or putting them to death. (p. 4)

The solution to school violence is not the further curtailment of student rights, but instead the development of programs and policies aimed at the real causes of violence—these causes are largely found outside the school system. They include a cultural tradition of endorsing violence as a solution to problems, the media's overemphasis on violence in programming and the news, and weak gun-control laws.

One of the most cost-effective strategies to protect children from violence is to expand after-school programs (Donohue, 1999). Studies report that enriched, recreational-based after-school programs are an excellent strategy for preventing juvenile delinquency. By providing after-school programs, the safety of children will be enhanced.

Gun sales must be restricted (Donohue, 1999). Little can be done to stop child-shooting deaths that most often occur outside of school grounds until the sale of guns is curtailed. Laws that reduce the sale of guns to adults will help limit the access of children to guns. Massachusetts and Virginia have implemented restricted gun sale programs that have dramatically reduced the number of juvenile homicides in each of these states (Donohue, 1999).

The media and news service organizations are doing a great disservice to American society through the growing emphasis on school violence. In a free society it is critical to inform the public about the homicides in schools. Media hype, however, has done a great disservice because it has led policymakers to believe that school killings are a growing social problem (Donohue, 1999). Donohue (1999) argues that public discourse aimed at a more objective understanding of school violence would greatly help the public's understanding of youth crime.

Alexander and Curtis (1995) suggest that programs aimed at enhancing teachers' understanding of school violence would also be helpful. Teachers need to realize that school violence is unlikely in the classroom and that this notion should be conveyed to students. Teachers should also realize that certain discipline techniques can help limit the potential for violence. For example, using behavior techniques that involve the child's family appears to be an effective approach for dealing with troubled children. The use of corporal punishment on disruptive students only enhances the possibility of violence. Teachers, like the public in general, must be aware that the potential for violence is much greater outside the school than within. The solution to violence is enlightened programs and policies based on fact, and not media hype. Sound public policy in the area of youth violence will help to protect students from violence as well as protecting their rights.

CHILD MALTREATMENT PREVENTION AND THE SCHOOLS

For over three decades, it has been recognized that closer linkages between schools and child welfare agencies would improve services to children and families (Downs et al., 2004). Human service programs have been conducting innovative school-based services for many years. Schools are addressing vexing challenges facing youth, families, and communities today (Downs et al., 2004).

Schools are involved in the prevention of maltreatment and family support programs. Schools are a primary source of reports of child maltreatment to child protection agencies, and educators are mandatory reporters in every state (Downs et al., 2004). Many child protection agencies are experimenting with placing social service workers in the schools to work collaboratively with school personnel on prevention and early identification of child maltreatment. Prevention efforts aimed at children are often conducted in schools and during after-school programs. These programs frequently include elements aimed at prevention of delinquency, substance abuse, and other unhealthy behaviors (Downs et al., 2004).

Increasingly, family support and developmental programs are linked to the schools. Downs and colleagues (2004) report that 5,000 school-based family support programs are currently in existence. These programs are characterized by the strong partnerships they form with schools and the mutual responsibility for outcomes (Downs et al., 2004).

The "school of the twenty-first century" concept was developed by Edward Zigler, one of the architects of the Head Start program. The concept eliminates the distinctions among family support, child care, and education, recognizing that learning begins at birth and occurs in many settings. The comprehensive program envisioned by this concept includes parent outreach and education, preschool programs, before- and after-school programs, health education services, networks for child care providers, and strong community support and involvement (Downs et al., 2004). This model of family support and prevention is currently being implemented in communities across the United

States, although it has not yet received a comprehensive evaluation (Downs et al., 2004). Although various initiatives linking schools, maltreatment prevention, and family-support programs show promise, the potential for collaboration between child welfare and school service systems has yet to be realized. A major challenge for the new century is to find effective strategies of collaboration for two of the major public service systems for children and families, the schools, and the child welfare system (Downs et al., 2004).

CHILDREN WITH DISABILITIES AND SCHOOL RIGHTS

Extending rights to children with disabilities in schools is a recent phenomenon in the United States. As mentioned earlier, important laws related to these rights include IDEA, Section 504 of the Rehabilitation Act of 1973, and the ADA. Activists who lobbied for the passage of laws protecting the rights of children with disabilities in the school setting grounded their arguments in *Brown v. Board of Education* (1954). The following statement from *Brown v. Board of Education* is often used by advocates for promoting the rights of children with disabilities in schools and American society:

> Today, education is perhaps the most important function of state and local governments. Compulsory school attendance laws and the great expenditures for education both demonstrate our recognition of the importance of education to our democratic society. It is required in the performance of our most basic public responsibilities, even service in the armed forces. It is the very foundation of good citizenship. Today it is a principle instrument in awakening the child to cultural values, in preparing him for later professional training, and in helping him to adjust normally to his environment. In these days, it is doubtful that any child may reasonably be expected to succeed in life if he is denied the opportunity of an education. Such an opportunity, where the state has undertaken to provide it, is a right which must be made available to all on equal terms. (p. 1)

The laws protecting children with disabilities in public schools mean special needs children can no longer be segregated from able children. Furthermore, the practice of excluding children with disabilities from schooling or providing them with grossly inappropriate education is a violation of the law.

The Education of All Handicapped Children Act of 1975

Two historical cases brought about the passage of The Education of All Handicapped Children Act (now titled IDEA). One was the *Pennsylvania Association for Retarded Children (PARC) v. Pennsylvania* (1972), which helped create equal protection and due process for children with disabilities. The second case, *Mills v. Board of Education* (1972) resulted in a federal district court ruling that children with disabilities must have access to schooling and a free, appropriate education.

IDEA makes certain funds available to schools if they comply with the requirements of this law. Section 504 of the Rehabilitation Act of 1973 also cuts off any and all federal funds from schools that discriminate against the disabled. If a school does not comply with IDEA, the federal government can also withhold federal funds to the school.

General provisions of IDEA were offered earlier in this chapter; more detailed provisions of IDEA are as follows:

1. Prior written notice must be given within a reasonable time before any proposed change in the child's educational program.
2. All notices must be written in "language understandable to the general public" and in the primary language of the parents. If parents are not able to read, the notice must be given orally or by other means.
3. The testing of children must be nondiscriminatory in language, culture, and race.
4. Children have a right to free, independent testing and evaluation.
5. Parents must have access to the records relevant to their child's case, and they have the right to have records explained and to make copies. If parents feel the records are inaccurate, they have a right to a hearing on the issue if the school refuses to amend the records.
6. Parents of children with disabilities have a right to a fair and impartial hearing concerning issues related to their child's education. Parents can be represented by an attorney.

7. The student has a right to remain in a current placement until due process proceedings are completed concerning the child's case.
8. A "surrogate parent" can be appointed for children with disabilities who are wards of the state or whose parents are unknown or unavailable.
9. Children's records are confidential. Parents may restrict access to the records of their child. Parents must be informed before any information in a child's file is destroyed, and they also have a right to be told to whom information has been disclosed.

Constable, Shirley, and Flynn (1996) summarize six rights under IDEA:

1. The right to attend school—the principle of *zero reject*. Each school-age person with a disability has the right to be educated in a system of *free, appropriate, public education* (FAPE). Agencies and professionals may not expel or suspend students for certain behaviors or without following certain procedures; they may not exclude students on the basis that they are incapable of learning; and they may not limit students' access to school on the basis of their having contagious diseases.
2. The right to a fair appraisal of their strengths and needs—the principle of *nondiscriminatory evaluation*. Socioeconomic status, language, and other factors need to be discounted and must not bias the student's evaluation. Decisions need to be based on facts: on what students are doing and are capable of doing in relation to behavioral outcomes individualized for the student. The resulting education would remedy the student's impairments and build on strengths.
3. The right to a *beneficial experience* in school—a principle of FAPE—means that schools must individualize each student's education, provide needed related services, engage in a fair process for determining what is appropriate for each student, and ensure that the student's education indeed confers a benefit. Education must have a positive outcome for each student. The emphasis of this discussion is not simply on provision of access to education but on adapting the system and on building capacities in the person with a disability so that certain results are attained.

4. The right to be *included* in the general education curriculum and other activities—the principle of the *least-restrictive environment*—means that the schools must include the student in the general education program and may not remove a student from it unless the student cannot benefit from being in that program, even after the provision of supplementary aids and services and necessary related services.
5. The right to be treated fairly—the principle of *procedural due process*—means that the school must provide certain kinds of information (notice and access to records) to students, special protection when natural parents are unavailable (surrogate parents), and access to a fair hearing process.
6. The right to be included in the decision-making process—the principle of *parent and student participation*—means the schools must structure decision-making processes in such a way that parents and students have opportunities to affect meaningfully the education the students are receiving. A related principle of enhanced accountability to pupils and parents is moving in the direction of report cards related to individualized goals and educational programs.

Even though parents and their children with disabilities have extensive protections under federal laws such as IDEA, it is not unusual for school districts to violate these laws. What this means is that parents of children with disabilities must make a concerted effort to understand their rights under the law and, in particular, to learn advocacy skills. Chapter 5 will focuses on advocacy strategies for parents and child advocates.

ADA and Rights of Children with Disabilities in Schools

The ADA is based on the human rights philosophy. It is grounded in the position that people with disabilities have not received the same treatment as others and that it is the responsibility of the federal government to affirm or reaffirm those rights through judicial and legislative actions (Pardeck, 1998). The humanitarian philosophy also underpins the ADA because people with disabilities are viewed as having intrinsic worth and dignity. However, a utilitarian view is also reflected in the ADA; for example, schools must make reasonable modifications to assist children with disabilities. Reasonable modifications include changing school policies, practices, procedures, and services offered. However, an educational institution can argue that a modification is unreasonable because of excessive costs. In other words, the cost of a modification for a child with a disability cannot necessarily outweigh the benefits. The utilitarian perspective always stresses the practicality and cost effectiveness of programs; the ADA takes a similar view on the issue of reasonable modifications (Pardeck and Chung, 1992).

Findings Supporting Need for the ADA

The ADA (Pardeck, 1998) was signed into law based on the following findings:

1. Forty-three million Americans have one or more physical or mental disabilities.
2. Historically, society has tended to isolate and segregate individuals with disabilities.
3. Discrimination in the areas of employment, housing, public accommodations, transportation, and education has been an incredible deterrent in the implementation of the rights of persons with disabilities.
4. Individuals who have experienced discrimination on the basis of disability frequently had no legal recourse.
5. Individuals with disabilities are intentionally excluded by architectural, transportation, or communication barriers and practices that result in lesser opportunities.
6. People with disabilities as a group occupy inferior status and are severely disadvantaged socially, vocationally, economically, and educationally.
7. Individuals with disabilities are a discrete and insular minority who have been faced with restrictions and limitations and subjected to unequal treatment.
8. The nation's proper goals should be to assure equality of opportunity, full participation, independent living, and economic self-sufficiency for persons with disabilities.
9. The continued existence of unfair and unnecessary discrimination denies persons with disabilities the opportunity to compete and costs the United States billions of dollars in unnecessary expenses resulting from dependency and nonproductivity.

Purposes of the ADA

Four purposes of the law, based upon the nine findings, are (Pardeck, 1998):

1. To provide a national mandate to eliminate discrimination against individuals with disabilities.
2. To provide an enforceable standard addressing discrimination.
3. To ensure that the federal government plays a central role in enforcing these standards.
4. To involve congressional authority in order to address the major areas of discrimination faced by people with disabilities.

Major Titles of the ADA

Title One: Discrimination Regarding Employment. No covered entity shall discriminate against a qualified individual because of disability with regards to job application procedures, hiring, advancement, discharge, training, compensation, or other terms of an individual's employment. A qualified person with a disability is someone who, with or without reasonable accommodation, can perform the essential functions of a position. Reasonable accommodation involves making existing facilities accessible, job restructuring, training materials, equipment, and modified work schedules. Discrimination because of a disability occurs when an employer with fifteen or more employees fails to make reasonable accommodation that would not cause undue hardship.

Title Two: Public Services. No qualified individual with a disability shall, by reason of such disability, be denied the benefits of services, programs, or activities of a public entity. For example, all public day care facilities must have accessible buildings for children and adults with mobility impairments.

Title Three: Private Accommodations and Services. No individual shall be discriminated against on the basis of disability in the full and equal enjoyment of goods, services, privileges, advantages, or accommodations by any person who owns, leases, or operates a place of public accommodation. Public accommodations would be places such as a hotel or other places of lodging; a restaurant, a theater, park, or zoo; and professional offices, schools, food banks, social services and day care.

Title Four: Telecommunications. Telephones must be available for those with speech or hearing impairments. Special emphasis is placed upon telecommunications relay systems, which allow for communication between parties, at least one of whom has a speech or hearing impairment.

Title Five: Miscellaneous. This section prohibits retaliation against an individual because of actions related to the act and charges various parties with preparation of plans, regulations and technical assistance manuals.

Unlike IDEA, the ADA covers both public and private schools. Title II of the ADA deals with state and local governments; public schools fall under these provisions. Title III covers public accommodations; public schools must also meet the mandates of this title. The purposes of both Title II and III are to integrate students with disabilities into school settings to the fullest extent possible and to provide them with the same educational opportunities enjoyed by others.

The following section supplies information about what actions schools must take under the ADA to integrate students with disabilities. The actions barred by the ADA in school settings are emphasized. Much of this information can be applied to all levels of educational institutions, from primary schools through secondary schools. An effort is also made to distinguish the differences mandated by the ADA for treating students with disabilities in public and private educational institutions.

Actions Educational Institutions Must Take

The ADA guarantees the rights of students with disabilities in educational settings. The reader should note that IDEA is an extremely narrow law when compared to the ADA because it only covers certain educational programs and services. The ADA, unlike IDEA, literally affects every aspect of the educational environment.

The ADA has four basic standards that govern the treatment of students with disabilities (Morrissey, 1993):

1. The program, service, or activity, when viewed in its entirety, must be readily accessible to and usable by students with disabilities.

2. A person with a disability must be able to access and act on information about a program, service, or activity.
3. When evaluating students with disabilities, screening and testing procedures must be fair, accurate, and nondiscriminatory.
4. Students with disabilities must be able to participate in an activity, service, or program offered to other students.

The ADA does not provide educators with a simple set of requirements or rules; it is a very complex law. ADA concerns in an educational setting must be judged on a case-by-case basis; however, educational institutions must follow a number of basic guidelines under the ADA.

Integration and Accessibility

Schools must ensure that programs are offered in the most integrated setting for students with disabilities. This is only possible if the programs and physical facilities are accessible to students with disabilities.

Integration is mandated by the ADA even if modifications are needed to a program so that a student with a disability can enroll. If a modification to the program is not possible, a school must offer separate opportunities for the student; however, all other efforts must first be exhausted. Under Title II of the ADA, if an entity offers a separate program, the person with a disability can decline to participate in favor of the integrated program.

Integrating students with disabilities can require modifications in program policies and procedures. The ADA requires schools to make reasonable modifications to a program as long as they do not fundamentally alter the program or result in undue financial or administrative hardship (Pardeck, 1998). Reasonable modifications include the following:

1. Notifying potential students with disabilities that a range of services and programs is available to them, including filling out forms, obtaining modified textbooks, and telling them where to call for information.
2. Offering returning students with disabilities a chance to register for classes early so any special adjustments they need can be arranged before school begins.

3. Letting a student with disabilities take an exam at a different time or location than other students.
4. If a student with disabilities transfers to the school during the academic year and the class is not accessible, reassigning the class to a different room is required.
5. Letting students with certain kinds of disabilities, for example mobility impairments, leave the final period class early so they can safely board transportation before the rush of other students.
6. Training teachers about the types of modifications they can make to accommodate students with disabilities.

These are examples of modifications that would fundamentally alter a school program (Pardeck, 1998):

1. Waiving an entrance requirement to a course or activity when the requirement bears directly on the child's chance of success.
2. Putting a child with a disability in a class where he or she would require so much individualized attention from the teacher that it would substantially reduce the amount of instruction offered to other students.
3. Placing a child with disabilities in a class where the auxiliary aids that he or she needs or behavior that the student exhibits substantially affect other students' ability to learn.

Teachers have a right to expect students with disabilities to take exams and complete course requirements. At the same time, however, teachers should recognize that under the ADA it is a rare case where they can justify excluding a student with a disability from a class or program. In most cases, reasonable modifications can be made so students with disabilities can participate (Morrissey, 1993).

Even though the requirements for physical accessibility are not specified in the ADA, Pardeck (1998) provides examples of the intent of the law. One example is that a secondary-level student with a disability should be able to access at least one biology lab, but not necessarily all of the labs in the school. A second example is that at least one location should be accessible to all services offered by the school.

Carrying a child with a disability up or down stairs is not considered a method of achieving physical accessibility to a program. Carrying a child is only permitted in manifestly exceptional circumstances and is not an alternative to installing ramps or chair lifts. In cases where carrying is the only option, the persons carrying the child with a disability must receive formal training on the safest and least humiliating method (Morrissey, 1993).

What constitutes a reasonable modification for a public school may be considered unreasonable for a private school. According to the ADA, fundamental differences exist between the obligations of public and private schools (Pardeck, 1998):

1. If a classroom or service is not accessible to a student with a disability in a public school, the classroom or service will have to be moved to an accessible area. Private schools, on the other hand, may work within the constraints of a single site.
2. For a public school system, removing barriers for persons with disabilities does not necessarily mean unreasonable costs; however, such actions may be unreasonable for a private school. The degree of such modifications required of private schools must be reasonable. Public schools, on the other hand, must make such modifications unless doing so would create undue hardship.

One other important difference between public and private schools under the ADA affects cases in which a school official decides to deny access to a student with a disability because the modification would fundamentally alter a program or result in undue hardship. A public school official who makes this decision must put his or her decision in writing. Private schools are not required to do this (Pardeck, 1998).

Public and private schools can impose requirements aimed at protecting students' safety. Such requirements, however, cannot be based on fears and stereotypes concerning students with disabilities. The following are examples of safety requirements under the ADA (Morrissey, 1993):

1. A student with cerebral palsy should be allowed to participate on a swim team if the child can perform the required swimming strokes and qualifies for the team. How the student gets into and out of the pool may involve help from others, but this cannot be the basis for excluding the student from the swim team.

2. A student with a disability associated with high levels of fatigue may not be able to safely take a long bus ride on a field trip. Students with other kinds of disabilities, such as an emotional disability or learning impairment, usually do not pose safety risks to the self or others.
3. Most students with disabilities in primary schools cannot be denied access to a playground because of safety concerns.

Communication with Students with Disabilities

The communication requirements regarding students with disabilities under the ADA are very clear. These requirements include simple actions such as writing a brief message on a note pad for a hearing-impaired student to more complex actions such as providing a reader for a child who is blind.

The ADA puts two limits on what schools must do in the area of communication with students with disabilities. First, schools are not required to do anything that would fundamentally alter a program or result in an undue hardship. Second, a reasonable modification does not have to be the latest or most expensive technology. The following are general requirements concerning communication under the ADA (Morrissey, 1993):

1. Schools should give first consideration to the preference of a student with a disability when choosing which type of auxiliary aid or service to provide.
2. Telecommunication devices should be installed for deaf or hearing-impaired students.
3. Schools must ensure that students with disabilities, including those with vision and hearing impairments, are able to get information about the availability of services and the accessibility of facilities.
4. The international symbol for accessibility should be posted at the entrance of all buildings that are accessible.

The ADA also mandates that when a private school, for example, recruits students, children with disabilities must have the same opportunities as others to access information about the school's educational programs.

Testing Procedure

The ADA has a number of clear requirements that affect the testing process. The following are the general requirements that schools must follow in testing students with disabilities who need reasonable modification in this area (Morrissey, 1993):

1. A student with a disability may be given additional time to take a test.
2. The test may be read to a student with a disability.
3. A student with a disability may have to take a test at a different time and place.
4. The student with a disability may receive individualized proctoring during a test.
5. The student with a disability may have to use some other means to demonstrate knowledge or ability that may not be reflected in a standard test.

As indicated in this section, the ADA does set limits to the actions schools must take to accommodate students with disabilities. A general requirement under the ADA is that schools do not have to do anything that would fundamentally alter a program or service or cause an undue hardship for a school. However, the ADA does require that students with disabilities must be integrated into classes and activities with able students whenever possible. In most cases, it will be much easier to accommodate a student with a disability than to explain legally why the child was denied access to a program or school activity (Morrissey, 1993).

Actions Barred by the ADA

A number of actions are barred by the ADA. Many of these actions barred by the ADA are also prohibited under Section 504 of the Rehabilitation Act of 1973. In general, schools cannot do anything that discriminates against students with disabilities. The ADA permits denying access to a program or service in only a few, limited circumstances. As stressed earlier, it is much easier for schools not to discriminate than to later face a legal challenge. Keeping this point in mind, the following actions are barred under the ADA for both public and private schools (Morrissey, 1993).

Generalizations. Every decision that affects a child with a disability must be made on a case-by-case basis. For example, a rule stating that visually impaired children cannot participate in a program is probably a violation of the ADA.

Denial of Opportunity. A school cannot deny a qualified student with a disability the opportunity to participate or benefit from programs or activities offered by a school.

Unequal Opportunity. Schools cannot offer lesser opportunities to students with disabilities than those offered to able students. For example, a student with a disability has the same right to eat in a school cafeteria as do able students.

Separate or Different Opportunities. A school cannot provide a different or separate opportunity unless it can be determined that this modification is truly necessary. Schools must also determine if the adjustment can be provided in an integrated environment.

Right to Decline Separate or Different Programs. Schools cannot deny students with disabilities the opportunity to participate in services or programs along with other students, even if separate or different programs are available. Thus, schools cannot require qualified students with disabilities to take separate classes. This requirement enforces integration and choice for students with disabilities.

Right to Decline Special Aids or Services. Students with disabilities have the right to decline special aids and other services that are offered by a school. For example, they can decline special equipment offered by the school.

Use of Discriminatory Criteria. Schools cannot use criteria or methods of administration that discriminate against children with disabilities. For example, under the ADA a teacher cannot require that all assignments must be in writing; a student with a disability may have a right to demonstrate knowledge of a topic in a different format because of his or her disability.

Discrimination Through Eligibility Criteria. Schools cannot impose eligibility criteria that tend to screen out students with disabilities from programs or services. An exception to this requirement is allowed if the criteria are essential to the program or services offered by the school.

Surcharges. Students with disabilities cannot be charged for an accommodation or modification to a program. For example, if a student needs an interpreter, the school cannot charge the student for this service.

Discrimination Through Association. Schools cannot discriminate against a student because he or she has a relationship with a person with a disability. For example, a student cannot be denied admission to a school event because he or she is accompanied by a friend who has an emotional impairment.

Retaliation. Schools cannot take a negative action against an individual because he or she opposed a practice made unlawful by the ADA. This requirement protects both persons with disabilities and others who file complaints under the ADA.

Coercion. School systems cannot coerce, intimidate, threaten, or interfere with any individual who exercises his or her rights under the ADA. This companion requirement to retaliation covers persons with disabilities and others involved in exercising one's rights under the ADA.

Sharing Information on the ADA

Child advocates should work toward schools sharing information on the ADA with the public. Teachers in particular need to share information on the ADA with students with disabilities and their parents. Morrissey (1993) recommends the following strategies for disseminating information by teachers to both groups.

1. Course selection and career planning information should be available in alternative formats.
2. Students with disabilities who have questions about course selection or career planning are provided with the contact person with this information.
3. Students with disabilities are provided with information about special opportunities, events, and eligibility criteria for participating in a variety of ways.
4. All information about eligibility for programs has a contact person indicated.
5. All information about programs indicates if a response is required, from whom, when it is due and in what form, as well as the consequences of not responding.
6. Students with a known disability are asked how they prefer to receive and submit information.

7. School officials know about the personal information needs of students with disabilities and are responsible for ensuring that they receive information in a timely manner and a usable format.
8. Students with known disabilities receive information about programs in the format they prefer.
9. Students with known disabilities are permitted to respond to information about programs in the format they prefer.
10. If students with known disabilities do not respond to time-sensitive information, they are contacted again by appropriate means.

The following are helpful strategies for teachers sharing information with parents with disabilities:

1. All information sent home clearly indicates whom to call for answers to questions or concerns.
2. Parents with known disabilities are permitted to receive and submit information about school programs and services in the format they prefer.
3. School officials accommodate requests of parents with disabilities for alternative formats and methods of exchanging information.
4. School officials who know about the special information needs of parents with disabilities should be responsible for ensuring that parents receive information in a timely manner in the format they prefer, and when parents with known disabilities do not respond to time-sensitive information, the officials contact them again.

Complaints and Enforcement

The ADA is the broadest-based statute guaranteeing the rights of children with disabilities in schools. Even though the ADA is a complex law and has a far-reaching scope that affects schools in a number of ways, the complaint procedures are relatively simple to implement. These procedures build on Section 504 of the Rehabilitation Act of 1973; they also are similar to those found under Title VI of the Civil Rights Act of 1964. School officials who are familiar with the complaint procedures under Section 504 of the Rehabilitation Act of 1973 will find similar procedures under the ADA.

Schools have strong incentives to comply with the ADA because losing a complaint can be extremely costly. Public schools can lose their federal funds if found in violation of the ADA. Private schools can be required to pay actual damages and federal fines of up to $50,000 for the first offense and $100,000 for subsequent offenses. Also, both public and private schools that lose in court have to pay all attorney's fees (Morrissey, 1993). It is also important to note that students with disabilities or their caregivers who feel their rights or their child's rights have been violated under the ADA do not have to complete a local administrative proceeding before going to federal court. This is the case for both public and private schools.

Public Institutions. Complaints may be filed by persons who believe they have been discriminated against because of their disabilities. The individual or an authorized representative may file a complaint. Complaints may be filed with any federal agency, all of which must be forwarded to the U.S. Department of Education's Office for Civil Rights for review and investigation. A complaint must be filed within 180 days of the alleged discrimination unless the Department of Education extends the deadline. Once a complaint is received, the Department of Education investigates and attempts to resolve the complaint informally. If informal attempts fail, the department will issue a "Letter of Findings" that includes the following (Morrissey, 1993):

1. Findings of fact and conclusions related to the alleged violation.
2. A description of what the school must do to resolve each of the violations found.
3. A notice of rights available to the complainant, including the right to sue in federal court.

The Department of Education will also notify the Department of Justice and embark on formal negotiations with the school to try to achieve voluntary compliance. At this stage, any voluntary compliance that is agreed to must include the following (Morrissey, 1993):

1. It must be in writing and signed by all parties.
2. It must address each violation in the complaint.

3. It must specify the corrective action to be taken and a timetable for completion.
4. It must provide assurances that the discrimination will not occur again.
5. It must provide for the enforcement of the formal agreement by the attorney general.

If voluntary compliance efforts fail, the Department of Education must refer the matter to the attorney general with a recommendation for appropriate action. Such action can include the filing of a lawsuit in federal court and may also result in the termination of federal funds to the school after an administrative hearing (Morrissey, 1993).

Private Institutions. An individual with a disability can proceed against a private school under circumstances such as (1) if the person believes he or she has been discriminated against because of his or her disability or (2) if the person has reasonable grounds to believe that he or she is about to be discriminated against because of his or her disability. For example, the person might believe that blueprints or floor plans for alterations or new construction discriminate because they do not provide proper access to a school building (Morrissey, 1993).

In either circumstance, the individual can file a civil suit seeking preventive relief, such as a temporary or permanent injunction or restraining order. If the person filing suit requests it, the court can appoint an attorney to represent him or her. In addition, the court can permit the attorney general to intervene in the civil suit if the attorney general certifies that the case is of importance to the general public and larger society (Morrissey, 1993).

The court can order a wide range of injunctive relief if it finds the private school guilty of discrimination. The court can require the school to (Morrissey, 1993):

1. Alter facilities to make them readily accessible and usable by persons with disability.
2. Offer a service or modify a policy.
3. Provide alternative methods for the person with a disability to complete a task.

The court can also impose fines of up to $50,000 for the first offense and $100,000 for each subsequent offense and require the payment of actual damages to the complainant. The person with a disability can also ask that the attorney general investigate the alleged discrimination.

If a complaint is filed by a person with a disability against a public or private school, school officials should be able to document the following (Morrissey, 1993):

1. All students, including students with disabilities, are judged on the same standards.
2. All students, including students with disabilities who have the same qualifications and educational needs and interests, are offered the same educational opportunities.
3. If the need for accommodation arose, the staff and other school officials discussed options with the complainant.
4. The school officials offered reasonable and effective options and program modifications to the complainant.

If these steps can be documented, schools are in a strong position to defend any complaint. What this simply means in terms of organizational behavior is that all students should be provided the same educational opportunities regardless of disability and that the school can document that it has done so.

RECENT SUPREME COURT RULINGS ON THE ADA AFFECTING CHILDREN'S RIGHTS

Bragdon v. Abbott (524 U.S. 624 [1998]) resulted in an important ruling by the U.S. Supreme Court concerning persons who have HIV infection. The Court ruled that a person with HIV infection, even though it has not yet progressed to the so-called symptomatic phase, is disabled under the ADA. The Court also affirmed that patients infected with HIV posed no direct threat to the health and safety of dentists. One could generalize this ruling to health care providers in general (Pardeck, 2001).

In the *Bragdon v. Abbott* case, Sidney Abbott, an HIV-infected patient seeking dental treatment from Dr. Randon Bragdon in 1994, disclosed her HIV infection on the patient registration form. Dr. Bragdon refused to treat her in his office. He did, however, offer to perform the dental treatment needed in a hospital facility. Ms. Abbott refused the treatment and filed a lawsuit against Dr. Bragdon alleging that Dr. Bragdon's refusal to treat her in his dental office was a violation of her civil rights under the ADA. A Federal court ruled that Ms. Abbott was discriminated against by Dr. Bragdon under the ADA. In 1998, the Supreme Court upheld the lower courts' ruling (Pardeck, 2001).

During the summer of 1999 the U.S. Supreme Court attempted to help clarify the definition of a disability under the ADA. The cases involved in this attempt include *Sutton v. United Air Lines* (527 U.S. 471 [1999]), *Murphy v. United Parcel Service Incorporated* (527 U.S. 516 [1999]), and *Albertsons Incorporated v. Kirkingburg* (527 U.S. 555 [1999]) (Pardeck, 2001).

In *Sutton v. United Air Lines,* identical twin sisters were denied pilot positions on the basis of poor eyesight. Both sisters had 20/20 corrected vision and had considerable experience as commercial pilots with regional airlines. United Air Lines requires pilots to have at least 20/100 vision in each eye without any corrective measures. The sisters' claimed they were covered under the ADA, since without corrective measures their eyesight is poor enough to substantially limit a major life activity, seeing. The airline countered that because their sight is normal with corrective measures the sisters were not disabled under the ADA. A lower federal court ruled in favor of United Air Lines; in the summer of 1999, the Supreme Court upheld this decision (Pardeck, 2001).

Murphy v. United Parcel Service Incorporated involved Vaughn Murphy, who was a mechanic with United Parcel Service. Murphy began working for United Parcel in 1994. As a mechanic, Murphy was required to have a Department of Transportation (DOT) health card because he would need to drive large trucks for road checks. Murphy's initial physical exam cleared him and he was given a DOT health card and commercial driver's license. A month later, a blood pressure reading showed his blood pressure to be above DOT guidelines, and he was fired by United Parcel because of his blood pressure level. Murphy claimed he had a disability under the ADA because without medication he could not carry out major life activities. Murphy argued that United Parcel should allow him to adjust his medication in order to lower his blood pressure to a level acceptable to the DOT health guidelines as a reasonable accommodation. A lower court ruled in favor of United Parcel. The court held that Murphy was terminated because his blood pressure exceeded the DOT's requirement and therefore was not a qualified individual with a disability. In 1999 the Supreme Court upheld the lower federal court's ruling (Pardeck, 2001).

The third employment case involved *Albertsons Incorporated v. Kirkingburg.* In 1990, Kirkingburg, a truck driver, passed the necessary tests for a license despite limited vision in one eye. Kirkingburg was erroneously certified by the DOT and granted his commercial truck driver's license. When Kirkingburg was correctly assessed in 1992, he was told that he must get a waiver of the DOT standards under a waiver program begun that year. Albertsons, however, fired him for failing to meet the basic DOT vision standards and refused to re-hire him after he received a waiver. Kirkingburg filed a discrimination lawsuit under the ADA against Albertsons. A lower federal court ruled that Kirkingburg was not qualified without an accommodation because he could not meet the basic DOT standards and that the waiver program did not alter those standards. An appeals court ruled that Kirkingburg had established a disability under the ADA by demonstrating that the manner in which he sees differed significantly from the regulations in setting a job-related vision standard. Furthermore, Alberstons could not use compliance with the DOT regulations to justify its requirement because the waiver program was a legitimate part of the DOT regulatory scheme (Pardeck, 2001).

Albertsons Incorporated v. Kirkingburg was appealed to the U.S. Supreme Court, which reversed the appeals court ruling. The Supreme Court held that an employers' right to set safety guidelines or adhere to federal guidelines was seen as enough reason to refuse to hire or fire an individual. Furthermore, even if the DOT waived the sight guidelines on an experimental basis, employers do not have to waiver their safety standards (Pardeck, 2001).

In *Sutton v. United Airlines, Murphy v. United Parcel Service,* and *Albertsons Incorporated v. Kirkingburg,* the Supreme Court ruled against the plaintiffs. In *Sutton,* the Supreme Court found that whether an individual has a disability as defined by the ADA depends upon the effect of one's condition or impairment "in reference to the measures that mitigate the individual's impairment." In other words, people should be evaluated on the basis of their condition with the use of medication or assistive devices when determining whether their disability substantially limits major life functioning. The same line of reasoning applied to the *Murphy v. United Parcel Service* and *Albertsons Incorporated v. Kirkingburg* (Pardeck, 2001).

Olmstead v. L. C. (527 U.S. 581 [1999]) has far-reaching effects on disability services provided by state and local government. The plaintiffs in this case were two intellectually and emotionally impaired patients who were institutionalized in the state of Georgia. The plaintiffs claimed that they were denied services in the most integrated setting because they were placed in an institutional care. They claimed that institutionalization segregated them from the rest of society unnecessarily. The doctors for the plaintiffs found that community-based treatment was more appropriate for their conditions and treatment needs (Pardeck, 2001).

A lower federal court ruled in favor of the plaintiffs, finding that if the state confines an individual in an institutionalized setting when a community placement is more appropriate it violates a core principle underlying the ADA, that being to integrate persons with disabilities into the larger society. *Olmstead v. L. C.* was appealed to the Supreme Court; the Court ruled that the institutionalization of mentally disabled people is a form of discrimination and that the state of Georgia violated the plaintiff's rights under the ADA (Pardeck, 2001).

In 1998, George Lane and Beverly Jones brought a lawsuit against the state of Tennessee under Title II of the ADA alleging that several courthouses in the state were inaccessible to a person who uses a wheelchair. They filed suit under Title II, which prohibits governmental entities from denying public services, programs, and activities to individuals on the basis of their disability. In addition, it provides that persons who have been harmed by discrimination can seek damages from governmental entities, including the states. The Lane case raised an extremely important issue: Does Congress have the power to override the states' immunity from suit and authorize Title II plaintiffs to seek damages from the states? The Supreme Court ruled in favor of Lane (*Tennessee v. Lane*, 541 U.S. 509 [2004]).

Supreme Court rulings over the past several years have had a profound impact on the ADA. Specifically, these rulings have important implications for children's rights. Children who are HIV positive are protected by the ADA and cannot be denied services because of this medical condition. The rulings on the definition of disability may limit the rights of children in that if their condition with the use of medication or assistive devices corrects their disability and does not substantially limit major life functioning they may be protected by the ADA. The *Olmstead* ruling means children do not have to live in an institutional setting if it is determined that community-based care is better for the child. Last, the *Lane* ruling means that children who are denied access to a state government building do have recourse under Title II of the ADA. This ruling means that Title II still governs the behavior of state governments; many child advocates felt the Court would find Title II unconstitutional.

COMPARISON OF THE ADA AND IDEA

Table 3.1 provides a comparison of the ADA and IDEA. A thorough understanding of both laws will enhance the effectiveness of child advocates when working with children with disabilities in schools. It is noted that the requirements of Section 504 of the Rehabilitation Act of 1973 are almost identical to ADA requirements. The major differences between the two laws are that Section 504 applies to only public and private schools receiving federal money. Both public and private schools, regardless of whether they receive federal funds, are bound by the requirements of the ADA.

As can be seen in Table 3.1, all children with disabilities are covered under the ADA; however, a child's disability must fall into a certain category to receive protection under IDEA. Accountability is implemented differently under each law. The ADA is complaint driven; IDEA receives periodic monitoring from the U. S. Department of Education.

Table 3.1 also shows that a public school with fifty or more employees must conduct a self-evaluation of its policies and programs that potentially discriminate against students and others with disabilities. IDEA requires a three-year plan to be completed to ensure compliance. Both public and private schools must comply with the ADA; under IDEA, compliance is required only of schools receiving money for this program.

Table 3.1 presents the complaint procedures for both programs. Under the ADA, individuals who feel they have been discriminated against because of a disability can file a complaint with the U.S. Department of Education; complaints under IDEA must first exhaust all due process provisions before going to court. The definition of a disability under the ADA includes three prongs; IDEA identifies a dis-

TABLE 3.1. Comparison of Basic Elements of ADA and IDEA to Elementary and Secondary Education

Concept	ADA	IDEA
Scope and protection	Prohibits discrimination on the basis of disability in public and private schools.	Prohibits discrimination on the basis of disability in the provision of a free appropriate public education.
Accountability	Complaint driven.	Schools are subject to periodic monitoring and audits conducted by U.S. Department of Education.
Administrative requirements	Public schools with fifty or more employees must conduct a self-evaluation assessing the extent to which they discriminate in policies and practices concerning persons with disabilities. They also must include a plan for correcting problems identified.	State educational agencies must complete a three-year plan that ensures compliance.
Compliance	All public and private schools must provide services and opportunities to students with disabilities.	State and local educational agencies, and private schools under contract with such agencies, must comply.
Complaint process	Individuals who are discriminated against in services have two options: file a complaint with the U.S. Department of Education or sue in federal court.	Individuals must exhaust the due process procedures before going to court.
Definition of a disability	A student with a disability who has a physical or mental impairment, has a record of such an impairment, or is regarded as having an impairment. The impairment must substantially limit a major life activity.	A child between three and twenty-one who falls within a category defined as a disability under IDEA.
Federal enforcement agency	The U.S. Department of Education with the assistance of the U.S. Department of Justice.	The U.S. Department of Education.
Funding	No funding through the ADA. For-profit private schools can receive federal tax credits and deductions.	Funds are available through a formula grant program.

ability as falling within distinct categories that include but are not limited to intellectual impairment, learning disabilities, emotional disabilities, and other related disabilities. A child may be defined as having a disability under the ADA, but may not necessarily be considered disabled under IDEA. For example, a child may have a mobility impairment that qualifies him or her for protections under the ADA; however, the impairment does not necessarily mean the child needs special education services offered under IDEA.

The U.S. Department of Education plays a central role in enforcing both the ADA and IDEA. It can be observed in Table 3.1 that the ADA has no funding; funding is available for IDEA.

The following are the basic differences between the ADA and IDEA:

1. More children will be qualified as being disabled under the ADA than under IDEA. The ADA employs a very broad definition for defining a disability.
2. The ADA is complaint driven; IDEA receives periodic monitoring from the federal government.
3. Under the ADA, all public and private schools must provide students with disabilities the opportunity to participate in services and programs; IDEA covers only those schools receiving IDEA funding.
4. Under the ADA, one can file a complaint with the U.S. Department of Education or file a lawsuit in federal court. IDEA requires that all due process mechanisms be exhausted before filing a lawsuit.
5. Disability is defined differently under each law.
6. The ADA has no direct funding; IDEA is funded.

NO CHILD LEFT BEHIND ACT

The No Child Left Behind Act (NCLBA) was signed into law by President George W. Bush on January 8, 2002. The act made the largest changes to the federal education assistance program, the Elementary and Secondary Education Act (ESEA), since the inception of ESEA. The goals of the NCLBA are to ensure the funds spent by the federal government improve student achievement, implement annual assessments in reading and math in grades 3 to 8, increase greater accountability of teachers and improve teacher training, and to increase the focus on math and science in the classroom (Lunenburg and Ornstein, 2004).

Background of NCLBA

Improving the nation's K-12 education system is the top priority of NCLBA. H.R. 1 (The "No Child Left Behind Act") reauthorized the ESEA—the largest federal education program, providing about $26.5 billion (Fiscal Year 2002) in direct assistance targeted to low-income and minority populations. ESEA consists of fourteen separate titles. The House passed its version of H.R. 1 by a vote of 384-45 in May 2001. The Senate bill (S.1, the Better Education for Teachers and Students [BEST] Act) passed by a 91-8 margin in June, 2001. The Conference Committee (consisting of members of the House and Senate appointed by congressional leadership) negotiated the final bill language, which was passed by the House on December 13, 2001, by a 381-41 margin and the Senate on December 18, 2001, by an 87-10 margin. President Bush signed H.R. 1 (P.L. 107-110) on January 8, 2002.

Key Provisions of the NCLBA

The following list the key provisions of the NCLBA:

1. *Annual Assessments:* All states must implement annual tests in reading and mathematics in grades three to eight. Tests must be aligned to state academic standards. All students (95 percent) must participate, and the assessments must be the same for all students. Assessments measure gains in student achievement, and results must be compared from year to year within the state. By 2007-2008, states must administer science assessments at least once in each grade span from three to five, six to nine, and ten to twelve.
2. *National Assessment of Educational Progress (NAEP):* All states are required to participate in the NAEP for reading and math to verify results of state tests. The NAEP would be administered every two years in both reading and math to a sample of fourth and eightth graders. Costs for participating are covered by the federal government.

3. *Accountability:* All schools and school districts will be held accountable for all major student groups making "adequate yearly progress" toward being "proficient," as judged against state academic standards. Within twelve years, all students must be proficient. All major student groups (racial and ethnic minorities, students from low-income families, students with limited English proficiency, or students with disabilities) must make annual progress for schools and districts to succeed. Failure to make annual progress in two successive years would trigger aid for improvements. Persistent failure over the next three years would require additional improvements, progressively greater corrective action, and then complete restructuring.

4. *Data Disclosure on Results:* All school districts are required to disclose, by school, annual student performance data for every major student group in formats easily understood by parents and educators. Each state also discloses disaggregated data annually on student achievement by school district. State by state progress toward meeting proficiency levels is public. Disclosure began with the 2002-2003 school year.

5. *Teacher Quality:* In five years, states must have all teachers highly qualified in subjects they teach. Veteran teachers must have a BA and pass a state test or a highly objective, uniform state evaluation of proficiency. All new hires must have a BA and must demonstrate knowledge of core subjects on a state test.

6. *Math and Science Excellence:* A new initiative authorizes up to $450 million annually for math and science partnerships in the states. Partnerships combine state and local education agencies with higher education, business, and nonprofit organizations, such as research entities and museums, to raise student achievement in math and science. Priorities are set by local needs, but can include improving teacher qualifications, knowledge and skills, curriculum, instructional materials, and intensive professional development activities. A separate program under the National Science Foundation will target an additional $160 million to the states for a few innovative partnerships to experiment with and widely promote best practices.

7. *Technology:* H.R. 1 combines technology programs currently in the ESEA into a $1 billion grant program to integrate technology into education. Localities can use funds for hardware, software, access, teacher and student training, curricula development, online learning, and efficient uses in administration and data management.

8. *Early Reading:* All states will participate in a new $1 billion initiative for pre-K and grades one to three reading programs to ensure all children can read by grade three.

9. *Flexibility:* The number of programs under the act was reduced from fifty-five under current law to forty-five. States and local school districts are given the flexibility to shift diverse federal program funds to match local priorities and achieve results. With the exception of "Title I" money, which is targeted at economically disadvantaged students, states and localities can decide how to allocate up to 50 percent of all other funds distributed by formula.

10. *Alignment:* All states must have challenging academic standards in core subjects and can use funds in H.R. 1 to upgrade standards. Student assessments must be aligned to standards. Data must chart student progress in achieving standards. Teacher preparation and professional development must be aligned to the goals of student achievement. Accountability systems with rewards and sanctions must be aligned toward achieving standards. State plans must demonstrate this systemic alignment or a path toward alignment.

NCLBA and Children's Rights

As the impact of NCLBA legislation continues to unfold across the country, educators and child advocates face the difficult task of explaining how NCLBA hurts schools instead of helps them (Lunenburg and Ornstein, 2004). NCLBA is the current version of the longstanding federal ESEA, first implemented in the 1960s.

Many education reformers believe that NCLBA is a fundamentally punitive law that uses flawed standardized tests to label schools as failures and punish them with counterproductive sanctions. It must be transformed into a supportive law that actually promotes school improvement and makes good on the promise to leave no child behind.

The legislation must be reconsidered and rewritten, particularly in the areas of assessment and accountability.

Opinion polls suggest most people know little about NCLBA; however, key promises within the law have wide support. For example, the law authorizes the federal government to increase funding for the education of low-income students. It mandates that states eliminate the academic "achievement gap" that exists between different groups of students, paying particular attention to the progress of students who historically have not been well served. It also requires states, districts, and schools to find ways to educate all students successfully.

Such promises have played a key role in winning support for NCLBA from some political and civil rights groups who do not share the move toward privatization of public schools and the general hostility toward public education. Understandably, some child advocates and school reformers, long frustrated with the quality of education for poor students, viewed NCLBA as a potential tool to force schools to improve. Clarifying the reasons why NCLBA, as currently written, will be unable to fulfill its lofty promises is key to building a coalition that can force Congress to make changes in the law.

SUMMARY AND CONCLUSION

This chapter covers the rights of children in public and private school settings. When children enter schools, many of their constitutional rights are curtailed. Areas covered in the chapter include freedom of expression and speech, censorship, and privacy. Several court cases are presented that offer important rulings related to each of these areas. Particular emphasis is placed on the rights of children with disabilities in schools. Problems related to child maltreatment in schools and violence were offered, and NCLBA was discussed.

The laws affecting children with disabilities in schools are presented, with major emphasis on the ADA and IDEA. As suggested in the chapter, child advocates need to be aware of the rights of children with disabilities in schools. The greater the depth of the child advocate's understanding of these complex laws, the more effective the advocate becomes when trying to correct a violation of a child's rights under the ADA or IDEA.

The chapter offers the complaint procedures under the ADA for students with disabilities. The differences between the procedures used for public and private schools are covered. What should be clear from the procedures used to investigate complaints by federal agencies is that successful defense against complaints depends upon whether school officials can document that the school offered equal opportunity to students with disabilities.

Chapter 4

The Rights of Able Children
and Children with Disabilities
in Day Care Programs

The goal of this chapter is to cover the rights of children in day care settings and the need to improve day care for children and their families. Three forms of day care exist for young children in the United States. The most common is family or home-based care; 37 percent of children receive this kind of care in homes other than their own. Sitter care in the child's own home is the second most used form of day care by parents; 31 percent of children receive this kind of care. The third is group day care centers, which 23 percent of children experience on a daily basis (Westman, 1991).

One important children's rights issue related to day care is the low wages received by day care workers. In the 1990s the average group day care worker received only $11,000 a year (Karger and Stoesz, 2001). The annual turnover rate of providers was 40 percent. The turnover rate for family or home-based care was even higher (Gormley, 1990). This means that the continuity of caregivers for many children in day care settings is not present. Continuity of care is critical in children's lives in order for them to meet basic cognitive, emotional, and intellectual developmental needs. It is noted, however, that quality group day care has a neutral effect on middle-income children, but has a profound positive impact on children of low-income families (Pardeck, Pardeck, and Murphy, 1987; Downs et al., 2004). What this means is that quality group day care can generally meet the needs of children.

What follows is a discussion focusing on the basic rights of all children in day care settings. The chapter will also cover the rights of special needs in day care children under the Americans with Disabilities Act (ADA). It will be emphasized that the ADA does not necessarily cover all day care settings. It is important for child advocates to understand the circumstances under which the ADA is enforced for special needs children in day care.

THE DAY CARE SYSTEM

Within the United States, state governments regulate day care through their social services departments. These departments license and inspect both family or home-based day care and larger, group-based day care centers. Group-based day care regulations typically cover such issues as ratio of children to staff, space requirements, and training regulations for staff. Family or home-based day care regulations usually cover ratios and training requirements; these requirements are often less stringent than for group-based day care (Gormley, 1990).

Group day care settings include regulations for play group requirements, sprinkler systems, and liability insurance. Home-based day care normally must have a fenced backyard, fire extinguishers, and access to an emergency vehicle. As a general rule, state regulations are more developed for group day care settings than other kinds of day care programs. It appears that the rights and needs of children are probably better met in group day care programs than in other kinds of child care settings.

Day care regulations improve the quality of care for children. The ratio of children to staff is very important. Training and educational requirements for staff clearly increase the quality of the day care experience for all children. Rules that require the day care site to be inspected for safety-related issues are a must. These rules normally call for the inspection of the quality of the electrical and plumbing work at the day care site. In many states, virtually no safety requirements are in place for home-based day care (Gormley, 1990). This is obviously a major social problem in the United States.

Keeping these points in mind, the rights of all children in day care should include the following (Gormley, 1990):

1. A guarantee of health and safety for children.
2. Standards that promote the mental, physical, and emotional development of children.

3. Opportunities for physical and emotional development through play and other activities.
4. Standards that govern children and staff ratios.
5. Standards that cover safety requirements, including appropriate space for children to learn and play.
6. Standards that require staff to have appropriate training and education.
7. Regulations that ensure children are free from maltreatment.
8. Standards for meeting the nutritional needs of children.
9. Standards that promote the involvement of parents in the day care program.
10. Standards that include regular inspection of day care facilities by the state.

Westman (1991) suggests that day care in the United States has much to be desired when compared with other developed countries. Virtually all developed nations other than the United States have comprehensive child care programs guided by highly developed policies. Given the limitations of day care in the United States, child advocacy aimed at improving day care is critical. Westman (1991) argues that a number of day care constituencies must be recognized by advocates in order for them to be effective. These constituencies include employed parents who place their children in day care, day care development specialists who promote the professionalization of providers, and the day care industry itself. A major concern of this industry is marketing their services to parents. Their goal is to make a profit from their service; given this goal, the day care industry attempts to influence laws and legislation regulating day care.

DAY CARE
AND CHILDREN WITH DISABILITIES

In order to protect children with disabilities, the ADA has barred day care centers from a number of actions. Day care programs cannot do anything that discriminates against children with disabilities. Day care staff will find it is much easier not to discriminate than to later face a legal action (Fersh and Thomas, 1993). The following are actions barred under the ADA for both public and private day care facilities (Pardeck, 1998). These are identical to the actions barred by public and private schools covered in Chapter 3.

Generalizations

Decisions that affect a child with a disability must be made on a case-by-case basis. For example, a rule stating that children with diabetes will not be admitted to a day care program is a violation of the ADA.

Denial of Opportunity

A day care center cannot deny a qualified child with a disability the opportunity to participate in or benefit from day care programs or activities.

Unequal Opportunity

Day care centers cannot offer lesser opportunities to children with disabilities than are offered to others. For example, a child with a disability has the right to play outside with other able children unless it can be proven that such an arrangement is an undue burden on the facility.

Separate or Different Opportunities

A day care setting cannot provide a different or separate opportunity for a child with a disability unless it can be determined that this modification is truly necessary. A day care center must also determine if the adjustment can be provided in an integrated environment.

Right to Decline Separate or Different Programs

A day care program cannot deny children with disabilities the opportunity to participate in services or programs along with other children, even if separate or different programs are available. Thus, a day care facility cannot require qualified children with disabilities, for example, to eat meals in an area away from able children. This mandate enforces integration and choice for children with disabilities in day care settings.

Right to Decline Special Aids or Services

The parents of a child with disabilities have the right to decline special aids and services offered to their child by a day care center. For example, parents can decline special assistive technology or other accommodations offered to their child by a day care program.

Discrimination Through Eligibility Criteria

Day care centers cannot impose eligibility criteria that tend to screen out children with disabilities from their programs or services. An exception to this requirement is allowed if the criteria are essential to the day care center's programs or services.

Surcharges

A child's parents cannot be charged by the day care program for an accommodation. For example, if a child needs an interpreter as an accommodation, the day care program cannot charge the child's parents for this service.

Discrimination Through Association

A day care program cannot discriminate against a child because he or she has a relationship with a person with a disability. For example, an able child cannot be denied access to a day care program because the child's parent has a disability.

Retaliation

A day care program cannot take a negative action against a child or his or her parents because they opposed a practice made unlawful by the ADA. This requirement protects the child with disabilities and the child's parents who may file an ADA complaint.

Coercion

A day care program cannot coerce, intimidate, threaten, or interfere with any individual who exercises his or her rights under the

ADA. This companion requirement to retaliation covers children with disabilities and their parents, as well as others who exercise their rights under the ADA.

COMPLAINTS AND ENFORCEMENT
OF THE ADA

The ADA is the broadest-based statute of all disability laws guaranteeing the rights of children with disabilities. Even though the ADA is a complex law and has a far-reaching scope that affects nearly every facet of American society, the complaint procedures are relatively simple to follow and implement. These procedures are built on Section 504 of the Rehabilitation Act of 1973; they are almost identical to those found under Title VI of the Civil Rights Act of 1964 (Shapiro, 1993). Day care providers who are familiar with the complaint procedures under Section 504 will find similar procedures under the ADA (Pardeck, 1998).

Day care programs have strong incentives to comply with the ADA, because losing a complaint can be costly. Public day care programs receiving federal funds can lose this support if found in violation of the ADA. Private day care programs can be required to pay actual damages and federal fines for violating the ADA. Both public and private day care programs that lose in court may have to pay all attorney's fees. It is important to note that parents who feel that their child's rights or their rights were violated under the ADA do not have to initiate or complete a local administrative proceeding before filing a lawsuit under the ADA. This standard governs both public and private day care programs.

Public Day Care

If the parents of a child with a disability feel their child's rights or their rights were violated by a public day care facility, a complaint can be filed under Title II of the ADA. The U.S. Department of Justice is responsible for investigating complaints filed against public and private day care programs. Once a complaint is received, the Department of Justice investigates and attempts to resolve the issue on an informal basis. If the informal efforts do not work, the department will issue a "Letter of Findings" that includes (Pardeck, 1998):

1. Findings of fact and conclusions related to the violations under the ADA.
2. A description of what the day care program must do to resolve each violation found.
3. A notice of rights available to the complainant that includes the right to sue in court.

Private Day Care

Discrimination complaints against private day care programs can be filed under Title III of the ADA. One circumstance for filing a complaint under Title III is when a parent feels his or her child with a disability has been discriminated against by the private day care provider. Another circumstance would be if the parent has reasonable grounds to believe that his or her child with a disability is about to be discriminated against. For example, the parent believes that blueprints or floor plans for alterations of a day care facility or new construction of a day care center do not provide appropriate access for a child with a mobility disability (Pardeck, 1997). When day care providers modify or change a day care setting, they must be sure that the modifications ensure accessibility.

Parents who believe that a private day care facility has violated the ADA may file a civil suit seeking preventive relief, such as a temporary or permanent injunction or a restraining order. If the person filing suit requests it, the court can appoint an attorney to represent him or her. In addition, the court can permit the attorney general to intervene in the civil suit if the attorney general certifies that the case is of importance to the public (Pardeck, 1997).

The court can order a wide range of injunctive relief if it finds the day care program did discriminate against the child with a disability (Pardeck, 1997). These include:

1. Alter the day care facilities to make them readily accessible and usable by children with disabilities.
2. Provide that the day care facility must offer a service or accommodation for a child with a disability.
3. Order the day care program to provide alternative methods for children with a disability to participate in day care activities.

Defending Against a Complaint

If a complaint is filed against a public or private day care program, the program should be able to document the following (Pardeck, 1998):

1. All children in the day care program, including children with disabilities, are judged on the same standards.
2. All children in the day care program with the same qualifications are offered the same opportunities.
3. If the need for accommodation arose, the day care staff discussed options with the complainant.
4. The day care program offered reasonable and effective options to resolve the complaint.

If these steps were taken and documented, the day care facilities should be in a strong position to defend against a complaint. What this means in terms of organizational behavior is that all children should be provided the same opportunities, regardless of whether they have a disability or not, and that the day care program documents that it has done so.

CHILDREN WITH DISABILITIES AND ADMISSIONS TO DAY CARE

A day care program cannot deny a child admission to a facility simply because the child has a disability. However, when considering admission, a day care program may assess the needs of a child with a disability and balance those needs against the day care facility's budget, staff, and other legal factors. The ADA is not intended to impose unreasonable demands on small day care programs. It should be recognized, however, that most of the accommodations needed by children with disabilities in day care are inexpensive. More often than not, an accommodation only requires a change in policy, procedure, or attitudes that cost the program very little or nothing.

What is critical for day care staff who decide not to admit a child with a disability is to base the decision on objective criteria. If this is done, it is legal to deny the child with a disability admittance to a day care facility. The following four standards allow for this action (Pardeck, 1997):

1. If a child with a disability's admission to a day care program fundamentally alters the nature of the program and no reasonable accommodation can be made, the child can be denied admission.
2. If the needed accommodation imposes an undue burden on the day care program, and no other reasonable accommodation is available, the program can deny the admission.
3. If accommodating the child with a disability requires an architectural change that is not readily achievable, it is legal to deny admission of the child.
4. The ADA does not require admission to a facility when a child with a disability poses a direct threat to the health and safety of other children, staff, or the child with a disability.

Day care programs cannot have a blanket admission policy that denies children with certain kinds of disabilities. Each case must be assessed on an individual basis. The following quote summarizes this standard (Child Care Law Center, 1995):

> A provider has an obligation to attempt to take the necessary steps to accommodate the special needs of a child with a disability before denying care to that child. For example, a provider may not refuse care of a child who has a mobility impairment simply because that child has a mobility impairment. The provider is required to assess the special needs of that child and attempt to find reasonable means to accommodate those needs. (p. 81)

However, if a child's disability is so severe that a small day care facility simply cannot provide the needed accommodation, this would probably be an undue burden under the ADA. A larger day care facility with greater resources may have to make the needed accommodation for the child with a disability because it would be more difficult to argue that the accommodation is an undue burden (Pardeck, 1997).

Reasonable Accommodation in a Day Care

When deciding to admit a child with a disability to a day care facility, a decision must be made about whether it is possible to care for the child in a way that is reasonable for the facility. Since each case must be judged on its own merits, a day care program that cannot care for a child with a severe disability may be able to accommodate a child with a milder disability. Reasonable accommodation for a child with a mild disability might be incorporating activities into a program that allow the child to participate in those activities or simply assuring that the child has access to the facility (Pardeck, 1997).

If an accommodation requires changing policies, practices, or procedures that do not fundamentally alter the nature of a day care program, the accommodation would be considered reasonable. Changes that would be unreasonable include those that create a health or safety risk for the child with a disability or others, or if the change imposes an undue hardship. The following provides guidance for what a fundamental alteration of a day care program entails (Child Care Law Center, 1995):

> A fundamental alteration of the program is a very high standard that is difficult to meet. It requires you to push beyond feelings of discomfort, reluctance, or inconvenience, and to make an honest assessment of what degree of change and accommodation are possible without stressing your program to the breaking point and without becoming unreasonable.
>
> Because this standard is so high, it is likely that programs of all sizes will be required under many circumstances to change their policies, practices, or procedures when necessary to integrate children with disabilities. If proposed changes in policies, practices, or procedures will fundamentally alter the nature of your program, you will need to consider whether any reasonable alternatives are available. (p. 82)

Guidelines for Determining an Undue Burden

In order to decide if an accommodation is an undue burden, this decision must be based on the circumstances of the day care program. An undue burden is defined as a significant difficulty or expense. The following provides guidance for determining whether an accommodation is an undue burden (Child Care Law Center, 1995, p. 83):

1. The cost of the proposed accommodation.
2. The day care program's financial resources.
3. The number of staff employed by the day care program.
4. The legitimate safety requirements of the day care program.
5. If the day care program is owned by a larger corporation, the overall financial resources, size, and location of the parent corporation are taken into consideration.
6. If the proposed accommodation imposes a significant difficulty or expense, and whether reasonable alternatives exist that do not impose an undue burden on the day care program.

Larger day care facilities will have greater obligations under the ADA than smaller ones. This means it is more difficult to prove an accommodation is an undue burden for larger day care programs than smaller ones.

An ADA Day Care Discrimination Case

An example of a discrimination case in day care involves a diabetic child and KinderCare Learning Centers. This case illustrates how the ADA is interpreted with a large provider of services.

The American Diabetes Association and the Justice Department filed suit against KinderCare, arguing that KinderCare violated Title III of the ADA because it discriminated against children with diabetes (Pardeck, 1997).

The lawsuit was brought by the American Diabetes Association on behalf of Jesie Suthard, a diabetic child, against KinderCare because the provider excluded children with diabetes and refused to provide assistance in blood glucose monitoring and other essential activities to the management of diabetes. As part of the settlement, KinderCare had to revise its discriminatory practice and change its national policy regarding children with diabetes. KinderCare was ordered to monitor blood sugar levels of diabetic children in their programs, diet and exercise must now be considered, and parents are to be alerted when glucose levels fall outside the appropriate, agreed-upon range (Pardeck, 1997).

What the KinderCare lawsuit means to day care providers is that they have important obligations under the ADA. It also provides insight into what a reasonable accommodation may be for a child with a disability in a day care facility. The settlement also suggests that day care programs have a very high standard to meet if they claim an accommodation results in an undue burden for a program. It is noted that KinderCare is a national provider; thus its obligation to children with disabilities under the ADA is greater than smaller day care providers (Pardeck, 1997).

RESEARCH ON THE EFFECTS
OF DAY CARE ON CHILDREN

Rising rates of maternal employment have resulted in a dramatic increase in the use of out-of-home care, particularly day care settings, for infants and young children. Whether one sees this trend as positive or negative, potentially reversible or here to stay, it is a demographic reality of tremendous import. Regardless of these trends, one of the concerns about day care is the effect it has on child development. The following summarizes the effects of day care on the emotional and social development of children (Downs et al., 2004).

1. For children of advantaged backgrounds, studies have found no differences in intellectual development, as measured mainly by standardized tests, between home-reared children and those experiencing day care. For high-risk children (i.e., those from low-income families), day care appears to have a positive impact on their intellectual development.
2. With a few exceptions, studies have not found major differences in mother-child attachment between children reared at home and those reared in day care. This suggests that day care does not have a negative impact on a child's emotional development.
3. Day care appears to affect a child's social development. Compared to home-reared children, those children experiencing day care seem to be more peer oriented and less likely to interact with adults. Behavioral differences related to less aggression and assertiveness, and to more cooperation have also been found between home-reared and day care children.

4. A few studies suggest that day care may have a positive impact on the family system in terms of family income and several other significant areas.

POLICY IMPLICATIONS

It must be remembered that research findings have social implications. Underpinning the findings on the impact of day care on children a distinction must be made between custodial and developmental day care. Specifically, the benefits that accrue to those who are enrolled in day care are available only in high-quality programs. If programs offer only minimal activities, they are nothing more than glorified babysitting services. As noted by a number of authors, these types of day care centers instruct children to be passive through routinizing their curriculum (Downs et al., 2004). True education, instead, requires that a challenging and enriched environment be provided for children on a regular basis.

In order to ensure excellence among day care facilities, however, adequate funding must be available for these programs. Throughout the history of day care, this has not been the case. Many writers blame this situation on the sexist character of society (Downs et al., 2004). That is, if women are conceived to be merely secondary workers, then the need for expanded day care services is by definition marginal. Clearly this sentiment was centrally important to President Nixon's veto of the Comprehensive Child Development Act in 1972.

Conservative economists have a penchant for believing that women do not work out of economic necessity. Instead, they contend that workforce participation is the result of freely choosing among numerous alternatives, one of which is to work. In this case, it is no wonder that the presence of women in the workplace is considered to be temporary, and therefore does not necessitate any serious policy changes with respect to family life. Contrary to this misconception, the majority of women who work outside of the home do so to assure the economic survival of their families (Westman, 1991). Thus, serious decisions must be made about future child caring practices. Particularly, significant improvements will have to be made in terms of funding day care or many of the current problems, such as sexual abuse of children in day care centers, will become commonplace.

Day care, in short, can no longer be viewed as a luxury. Since many mothers of young children must now seek work, overall shifts in our social priorities must be undertaken. Day care is no longer a personal but a political issue. What this means is that social decisions about women working must be made on the basis of social values. The fact is that an economic "reality" is shaping women's attitudes toward work, and thus their changing views toward economic survival must be given appropriate political consideration. Unfortunately, the current national government, along with its conservative economic attitudes, is out of touch with the economic state of American families.

Short of a complete restructuring of society, the following policy considerations must be implemented or quality day care will not be available to family systems in which both parents work.

Funding

The recent budget cuts have decimated the budgets of many social service programs, and day care is no exception. Therefore, money for salary increases and the training of day care workers is not available. The annual wages of day care workers during the past decade was about $11,000 (Downs et al., 2004). Such low salaries tend to repel educated, conscientious workers. This situation may place children in day care at risk.

Increased taxes for the general public, however, is not necessarily the only remedy for this situation. Quite frankly, only a limited amount of resources are available, which suggests that current fiscal priorities may have to be reexamined. Although many persons have an aversion to reallocating funds that are earmarked for the military, the present economic "reality" dictates that this is imperative. That is, if economic reasons mandate that most family members must work, then social solutions to the resulting problems must be sought. Consequently, in order to avoid further cutting of social services that are already inadequate, nonsocial programs might have to be trimmed. This is essential if day care workers are to receive proper training and wages, so that children are placed in comprehensive programs (Downs et al., 2004).

In addition, giving tax rebates to those who can afford to pay for day care is not an appropriate method for funding this service. Stated simply, such tax rebates assume that everyone has the ability to pay their children's matriculation fees. Policies that are based on this assumption are ineffective for two reasons. First, low-income persons are not assisted by this procedure; second, the rebate that is received by moderate-income families is not sufficient by itself to fund day care at a proper level. Only through a social, as opposed to an individual, policy can an equitable funding strategy for day care be extended throughout our society. However, taxation and budget reallocations are not the only sources of funding for day care.

Workplace

Employers must become increasingly involved in offering day care facilities. In order for this to take place, however, this service must be viewed as more than merely a fringe benefit, which employers may or may not elect to provide. Instead, workers must be understood as creating social wealth. Following this shift in thinking about work, both male and female employees have the right to demand day care services as part of the remuneration they receive for their labor. For if an economic "reality" determines the rate of participation in the labor force, then the products of work should be channeled toward meeting the needs of workers. Most important, this approach to funding social services is predicated upon socially created wealth, as opposed to private philanthropy. This allows women, along with workers in general, to have more control over their lives.

In terms of a family policy, this approach to organizing day care allows fathers and mothers to remain in close proximity to their children. This does not, however, imply that the traditional images of the family and the female worker are being surreptitiously resurrected, thus requiring that women fill their traditional roles. Rather, because work and the process of allocating the fruits of labor are democratized, women are able to participate fully at the workplace and in any family arrangement that may be chosen. Yet without democratizing work, day care will only be implemented as part of a policy of securing cheap female labor through tethering women to roles which underutilize their talents (Westman, 1991). A clear example of this was witnessed during World War II, when most factories had day care services, yet neither women's work roles nor their social position improved appreciably. In short, if women are viewed as creating a country's wealth through their labor, then it only makes sense that they must share equally in terms of how these products are distributed.

This is possible, however, only when social wealth is used to facilitate personal growth, such as allowing parents to work knowing that quality day care is available. When conceived in this way, day care is "normalized," or understood to be a legitimate right of every worker.

Labor Unions

Labor unions must also become more seriously involved in procuring this service for workers than in the past. Labor leaders, consequently, must change their current approach to contract negotiations. Specifically, they must begin to see themselves as caring for the social well-being of workers, instead of merely securing high salaries for union members. In other words, workers must be able to control the wealth that they generate, thereby enabling social institutions to reflect their needs. That is, salary increases may not be readily translated into improving the total quality of life for workers. This is because their wages only represent a small portion of the wealth which they actually produce. Unions, therefore, must demand that workers receive all the services their labor is able to support, which requires that organized labor alter its perception of the purpose of work. If work is understood to further a person's well-being, as opposed to generating only wages, then the outcome of this activity must be used to support workers' claims.

Bronfenbrenner (1970) notes that such an expanded conception of work begins to break down the distinctions that are typically made between play, education, productive work, and the roles traditionally assigned to men and women. In addition, when persons begin to recognize that their roles are intimately related to how they interact with their children and other family members, increased social integration is possible. Individuals are able to realize that any personal problem requires a global solution, one which promotes social solidarity. By promoting the idea that work is closely related to family life, unions may inadvertently correct the social fragmentation that is threatening the family system. This type of social unity, moreover, enriches both family and community existence.

Community Control

Local control of day care must be instituted. This means that those who use these services must be directly involved in their planning and organization. In the mid-1960s this type of proposal was quite common, yet community control of day care was a dismal failure. These programs failed, not because community members were disinterested but because their efforts were constantly frustrated by both local and federal bureaucrats. Community persons were invited to participate in organizational meetings until they began to take their newly discovered power seriously. Once they became too aggressive, they were hurriedly dismissed from their positions and excluded from any further involvement in community planning (Downs et al., 2004).

Many social activists argue that community members were easily intimidated simply because their initiatives were not sufficiently politicized. This approach to community activism can be successful only if it is understood against the backdrop of political disenfranchisement in the United States of low- and moderate-income persons. Individuals must be made aware that they have the right to be self-determining, while also recognizing that this ambition may be blocked by those who hold power. Community control, in other words, is often accompanied by a policy of social demoralization, and local control of services is not achieved. Because day care in general demands many social reforms, direct community participation in planning various approaches to this issue may stimulate the political awakening that is necessary for these changes to be inaugurated (Pardeck, 2002).

Changes for the Future

Changes must be forthcoming with respect to what is believed to be the functions of the family. Specifically, the family cannot be portrayed in the usual functionalist manner if day care is to flourish. According to functionalists, the family is supposed to be a microcosm of the larger society and reproduce its goals in children.

As functionalists note, the nuclear family is most appropriate for this undertaking. Yet overwhelmingly it has been documented that children who are enrolled in high-quality day care programs are more peer oriented, less fearful of authority, and more aggressive than is normally expected. In terms of the functionalist ideology, these are undesirable characteristics for families to be instilling in children.

Nonetheless, day care introduces an entirely new, democratic, or, as Habermas (1970) suggests, dialogical approach to socialization. The impact of this will certainly be experienced socially. This shift in socialization is commensurate with the general theme that underpins day care: the need to break with traditional role imagery. Accordingly, day care is a sort of double-edged sword, as it simultaneously opens society and makes new demands on the citizenry. Persons must be able to meet these challenges to traditional societal imagery for day care to survive.

In sum, day care raises many political issues which must be addressed in novel ways. The success of day care depends upon a correct apprehension of its political implications, so that appropriate supportive policies are formulated. Without such an understanding, this social program will be instituted without the necessary accompanying changes in social values, only to be undercut by traditional social structures.

SUMMARY AND CONCLUSION

The three common kinds of day care programs in the United States are family or home-based care, a sitter in the child's own home, and group day care. Of these, family or home-based day care is most common; group day care is the least common.

The regulations of day care programs vary from state to state. Group day care programs must follow the most detailed set of regulations; other kinds of programs have less-stringent regulations. This situation suggests that the rights and needs of children are better met for children placed in group day care programs.

The basic rights for children in day care include a right to safety, freedom from maltreatment, and being cared for by competent, trained staff. Given the fact that regulations vary from state to state, these basic rights are not always met for children in day care programs within the United States.

The requirements that public and private day care facilities must meet when caring for children with disabilities under the ADA are mandated under Titles II and III of the law. These titles help to integrate children with disabilities into day care programs.

The chapter offers steps for determining whether an accommodation is reasonable under the ADA and when an accommodation can be viewed as an undue burden. An undue burden is defined as an accommodation for a day care program that presents a significant difficulty or expense to achieve.

An ADA day care discrimination case is presented. The case provides insight into how the ADA worked to ensure that a large national day care provider must now provide accomodations for children with diabetes. This case suggests that day care programs have a very high standard to meet if they claim an accommodation is unreasonable. It also provides insight into other kinds of accommodations that day care providers may have to offer under the ADA.

Finally, the chapter explores the effect of day care on children's social and emotional development. A detailed discussion on the policy implications of day care is also presented.

Chapter 5

Children's Rights
and Residential Treatment

Patrick Morgan

Residential treatment settings for children are often staffed by various professionals, including social workers. In this kind of practice setting, practitioners offer critical services to juveniles; the families of these children are also typically part of the treatment plan. This chapter briefly reviews the history of the children's rights movement and the juvenile court in residential treatment. The major emphasis of the chapter explores the rights of juveniles in residential treatment and the strategies that professional staff must use to ensure these rights.

A BRIEF HISTORY OF RESIDENTIAL TREATMENT AND THE JUVENILE COURT

The history of children and youth in residential treatment is consistent with other areas of the children's rights movement. It is notable that the history of the juvenile court is tied to the development of residential treatment. The Illinois Juvenile Court Act of 1899 created the first separate court proceedings for adolescents. This was a result of a combined effort by the Chicago Visitation and Aid Society, the Waif's Mission, and the Chicago Women's Club. These organizations

---

Patrick Morgan currently resides in Fayetteville, Arkansas, with his wife and son. Mr. Morgan currently works as a therapist for sexually abusive youth. His other social work interests include the importance of spirituality in the healing of sexual, physical, and emotional trauma.

were inspired by Massachusetts' development of a separate probation system for juvenile offenders (Hawes, 1991).

The Illinois Juvenile Court Act possessed two components. First, it provided a special court for juveniles who violated a law or local ordinance. Second, "any respectful person" could inform the court if they had information about a child who was abused or neglected. Gradually, every state developed its own juvenile justice system.

The modern-day juvenile court system has developed a number of procedures aimed at protecting the rights of juveniles. The procedures used to protect the rights of the juvenile are different from those used to protect adults in the criminal justice system. For example, when a juvenile is charged with an offense, the child is referred to the juvenile court. This referral is done through a "petition" filed by the prosecuting attorney; the petition outlines the specific charges against the juvenile. Some states, including Alaska, Colorado, Michigan, Texas, Wyoming, and New Mexico, allow jury trials in juvenile cases; however, most states do not. The juvenile does have the right in all states to legal representation. Obviously, the legal process used to charge and convict an adult offender is much different than the process used by the juvenile court. Chapter 6 presents a detailed discussion of the procedures used to adjudicate the juvenile offender.

CHILDREN'S RIGHTS
IN INSTITUTIONAL SETTINGS

Institutional settings for juvenile offenders are designed to treat, not punish, juveniles. This difference is based on the premise that children are innocent beings who need to be guided and protected by adults. Society often perceives children as victims of dysfunctional family systems. Treatment in an institutional setting is designed to correct problems that are understood to be family based. This means that the family must be a part of the child's treatment plan. Juveniles in residential settings typically have indeterminate sentences. Indeterminate sentencing allows social workers and other professional staff to determine when the child has completed treatment. However, in some states, such as Missouri, judges are given the authority to order a determinate sentence when they feel it is in the community's and juvenile's best interest (Community Learning Center Division of Youth Services, 2000).

Judges usually place juvenile offenders in the physical custody of a state's youth service program. The role of youth services is to decide if a community-based program will be utilized or if the adolescent will be placed in a group home or other institutional setting. If the latter is decided, then it must be determined what kind of residential facility will best serve the juvenile's needs. Some states have different levels of security in residential settings; these levels normally include minimum, moderate, and secure care. The gender of the juvenile will be an important factor in determining the level of security for a child; most states have minimal alternatives of placement for female adolescent offenders.

The Placement Process

Each state has its own method for placing juveniles in residential treatment programs. Many factors are considered when deciding the level of security needed by a child who is placed in a treatment facility. These factors include the nature of the offense committed by the child, the age of the child, and the location of the treatment facility. An effective strategy for deciding the level of security a child needs is to use an empirically based measurement scale and the seriousness of the offense committed by the child. This strategy brings a degree of objectivity to the decision-making process and helps to eliminate possible favoritism.

However, sometimes using formal intake instruments will be antecedent to the rights of the adolescent offender. Zac's case is one example.

Zac, a fifteen-year-old male, was committed to a Midwestern state's Division of Youth Services for multiple assaults. According to the intake scale used, he was to be sent to a secure-care facility for nine months. The problem was that the facility was more than an hour away from Zac's home community, and his mother lacked the transportation to visit him on a weekly basis. Family contact needed to be maintained to help Zac succeed in treatment, especially since the treatment plan included the goal of returning Zac to his home.

The case manager advocated for Zac by writing his concerns on a special form summarizing the reasons why Zac should be placed in a medium-care facility close to his home. This recommendation, however, raised an ethical issue for the case manager. Specifically, was the case manager placing residential and professional staff in jeopardy by placing Zac in a medium-care facility? It is not unusual for professional staff in residential treatment to face these kinds of ethical dilemmas on a regular basis.

If a juvenile has received an indeterminate placement, the child has the right to know what he or she must do to be released from treatment. This can be accomplished in a number of ways. Some programs operate on a phase or level system and require the juvenile to be at a certain phase or level before a release can be earned. Each phase or level has a list of responsibilities and requirements that the child must meet. Often, it is the treatment team which decides if the requirements are met; even though this may seem subjective, measurements such as point systems or goal-attainment scales can be used as concrete measures for indicating treatment progress.

If a program does not have a phase system, then the individual treatment plan (ITP) is used as an indicator of treatment progress. The success of this approach depends on the cooperation between the treatment team, the adolescent, and the child's family. If the juvenile and family are not in agreement with the ITP, then obviously the motivation for change is lacking. To correct this situation, the family and adolescent must be involved in further development of the ITP. The following case illustrates how the child and family are engaged in the development of the ITP.

A Native American girl received an indeterminate sentence for property damage. She was very quiet and would not participate in group sessions. The treatment team believed that she needed to learn to communicate better with others. Her parents, however, saw this as an attempt to make their child into "someone that she was not" and reported that she was often quiet at home. The ethical dilemma in this case is how to engage the child while being respectful of the family's wishes and culture. The treatment team thanked the family for the information and explained that teaching their daughter coping skills would help her express her feelings and empower her to say "no" to her friends if encouraged to participate in illegal behavior or dangerous activities. The family knew and understood the reason for the approach and did agree that their daughter needed to learn better communication skills. The treatment team also learned more about the American Indian culture and how members of the family communicate with each other.

Medications

The use of medications in treatment raise a number of ethical issues for professional staff. One issue is the child's right of self-determination in the use of medications. Another concerns whether medication should be the core form of treatment or an adjunct to treatment received by a child. Some social workers view medications such as Ritalin or Prozac as unnecessary and even harmful—placing children in danger of further health risk. For some children, medications are a necessity for a successful treatment outcome. Even though self-determination is a critical concern, a child who refuses to take medications is violating the prescribed treatment plan. Side effects might also occur if the medicine is not taken on a specific time schedule.

Obviously, it is difficult to make a juvenile take his or her medications. Professional staff cannot physically force the child to take medication. One strategy might be to ask the child why he or she does not want to take medication. For example, the child may be experiencing some side effects or other forms of discomfort from the medication. Sometimes children do not like the idea of drug therapy because they feel a loss of control. This is particularly the case for juveniles who attempt to control interpersonal relationships. Another possible reason for refusing medication is that the child may feel that taking drugs means personal failure; that is, the child cannot control his or her own behavior.

Finally, every child in a residential treatment has a right to health care. This is very important, since some behaviors have biomedical causes. Taking care of an adolescent's physical needs also helps to build trust in the therapeutic relationship. A treatment team cannot meet the psychosocial needs of children unless, as suggested by Maslow, their basic physical needs are met first (Crider et al., 1986).

Specific Rights in a Residential Setting

The following is an excerpt from a handbook given to children placed in a group-home setting in a Midwestern state (Community Learning Center Division of Youth Services, 1999, pp. 4-6):

All youth in the care of the Division of Youth Services have certain rights and responsibilities that must be recognized. Youth have the right to grieve any violation of these rights through the grievance process. Youth have the right to:

1. Expect that they will be treated respectfully, fairly and will be addressed by name in a dignified manner.

2. Be informed of the rules, procedures and schedule which have an impact on them.
3. Not be subjected to corporal punishment, harassment, intimidation, threats, harm, assault, humiliation or interference with their physiological needs.
4. Not be discriminated against because of race, national origin, color, creed, sex or physical handicap.
5. Participate in religious services and religious counseling on a voluntary basis, subject only to the limitation necessary to maintain order and security.
6. Basic human needs and an overall safe environment maintained in compliance with state and local fire and safety laws.
7. Appropriate medical and dental treatment.
8. Have regular visits with family members and to send uncensored and uninspected mail. Incoming mail may be checked for contraband by staff in the youth's presence.
9. Wear appropriate personal clothing. This choice is limited relative to safety, security and hygiene.
10. Wear their hair and facial hair in any style they choose as long as it does not pose any health and safety problem.
11. The possession of personal items and jewelry. Any limitations imposed will be to maintain safety and security.
12. Participate in all available programs relative to their personal needs.
13. Participate in both indoor and outdoor recreation.
14. Report any problems or complaints they have without any fear of punishment.
15. Challenge any action in accordance with the appeal procedure.
16. Privacy from the media.

According to the principles of Maslow's hierarchy of needs, a resident will not be able to work on his or her personal issues until basic safety/security and physical needs are first met. The rights previously listed help to provide safety/security and physical needs for children; they also serve as a contract for children and their families in terms of treatment expectations. At times, however, professional staff will have to limit some of these rights if a child is acting out. For example, if a child threatens to leave treatment, professional staff may have to remove the child's access to certain activities as a form of discipline.

It should also be noted that some juvenile rights are up to the discretion of the treatment team. For example, whether or not a resident's clothing is appropriate is often a judgment call. To enhance the consistency of the treatment team, it is best that these issues are discussed in staff meetings so that all employees have a better understanding of what is expected of them. These expectations then can be better communicated to the children in treatment.

Grievance Procedures

Grievance procedures are readily available to adults in virtually every setting, including employment. These procedures help to ensure that policies are followed in a fair and equitable manner. Grievance procedures in residential settings help to ensure that policies are followed by professional staff. At times, however, children use the grievance procedures to get back at the treatment team or even to avoid addressing personal/family issues. In these cases, supervisory staff are usually involved to help process the situation and to ensure the child's rights are invoked, including the right to self-determination.

Self-Determination

According to the National Association of Social Workers' (NASW) code of ethics, each client has a right to self-determination. Social workers have the obligation to respect the client's choices, even if the worker believes it will result in negative consequences for the client. However, what about adolescents? Do they have the right to self-determination even though they may not be of the legal age of consent? Although these questions have no clear answers, everyone who works with youth, from parents to teachers, realizes that adolescence is a time of rebellion and exploration and often poor choices are made. The case of Jenny illustrates this point.

Jenny is a sixteen-year-old female who has decided to drop out of school and is not interested in a GED program. Her career plans include fast food, and she has expressed interest in exotic dancing. Obviously this juvenile is making choices that could very easily result in poverty, low self-esteem, and other dangers. In this case, the social worker and the treatment team gave Jenny an assignment on determining if she could purchase housing, transportation, and other items on a fast-food salary. To address the exotic dancing issue, she processed with her treatment group regarding why she finds that field appealing and was challenged to think of the negative consequences for that choice. Even though these interventions will not guarantee that Jenny will make better choices, it does allow her to see more options and possibilities.

Occupational Conflicts Within Residential Settings

Many different professionals provide services within residential settings, including nursing, psychology, education, criminal justice, recreation, and social work. Each occupation has its own treatment niche within the residential treatment setting. However, conflicts can occur due to the different treatment emphasis by each profession. For example, the strengths-based approach of the social work profession can conflict with the highly structured treatment approach used by the criminal justice professional. In reality, however, the treatment models stressed by both social workers and criminal justice professionals are critical to successful intervention outcomes. All clients need to learn their own strengths to improve their self-worth, but at the same time, structure and consequences are critical for teaching the consequences of chosen action. From a child's rights perspective, both treatment models appear critical to successful treatment outcomes in residential settings. Conflict among professionals can have a negative impact on service delivery. In residential treatment, it is imperative that professionals resolve these differences. The following guidelines from Kirst-Ashman and Hull (1999) offer a strategy for conflict resolution:

1. Gather information about the issues creating the conflict.
2. Determine if an ethical dilemma exists.
3. Determine the role of professionals in resolving the conflict.
4. Prioritize the most important issue for resolving the conflict.
5. When possible, share all relevant information with all persons involved in the conflict.
6. Examine the dilemma creating the conflict from a high level of moral reasoning.
7. Explore alternatives for resolving the conflict.
8. Weigh alternatives for each resolution.

9. Examine potential outcomes and consequences for various courses of action.
10. Determine a tentative resolution.
11. Propose the chosen resolution in the "court of professional opinion."
12. Consolidate.
13. Act.
14. Evaluate the results of the action.

When conducting conflict resolution, it is paramount that all parties have accurate, concise, and up-to-date information. Obviously, decisions made without all the facts and input from those affected by the decision will have negative consequences.

When disagreement exists over a child's treatment plan, it is helpful to use the problem-solving process to prioritize treatment goals. Loewenberg (1977) offers a strategy that may help professionals agree on the values that should guide treatment goals. These are as follows:

1. Protect life.
2. Maintain autonomy, independence, and freedom.
3. Foster equality of opportunity and equality of access.
4. Promote a better quality of life.
5. Strengthen every person's right to privacy/confidentiality.
6. Speak the truth and fully disclose all relevant information.
7. Practice in accord with rules and regulations voluntarily accepted.

These guidelines will help keep the welfare and well-being of the child as the most important treatment issue. Sharing information with the treatment team will also help practitioners gain insights into the child's situation and behavior from other professional viewpoints. For example, when consulting with a nurse, practitioners will gain a better understanding of the biological aspects of a problem such as bedwetting or, when consulting with a teacher, insight may be gained into the clinical aspects of a problem such as a learning disability. A critical role for social workers is attempting to combine the ideas of other professionals into a holistic perspective that enhances the assessment and treatment process.

Finally, the manner in which one advocates for a child must meet the standards of the "court of professional opinion." In other words, professionals must approve of the logic and methods used to advocate for a child. Disagreement among professionals is inevitable; it is critical, however, to resolve conflict in order to help ensure that the rights of juveniles in residential treatment settings are realized.

Education of the Treatment Team

The educational levels of staff working in residential treatment vary greatly. Entry-level positions usually require only a high school diploma, but a bachelor's degree in the social sciences is often preferred. Supervisory positions of frontline workers often require experience and a college degree. Case and facility management positions typically require at least a bachelor's degree.

One paradox of residential care is that the frontline staff (an entry-level position) often have the lowest educational requirement and receive the lowest pay when compared to the other positions. Workers who do not have appropriate training and education may not provide the best services to children. To improve service delivery, some residential treatment settings offer training focusing on communication skills, sexual abuse, and conflict resolution. It is also critical for frontline workers to have appropriate supervision.

Policy and Residential Care

National, state, and local policies have an effect on service delivery in residential treatment. An example of these policies is that in some states adolescent sex offenders must register with the local government where they live regarding their prior history. Even though these laws may provide public safety, they do have an impact on the duties and responsibilities of professionals in the residential care setting. For example, if a juvenile sex offender is on furlough or has been released from treatment, professional staff must ensure that the child is registered with local authorities and continues to have intermittent contact with the treatment facility. Other states may not have this requirement.

Practitioners must be familiar with all the policies that govern treatment intervention. As many practitioners realize, policies from different levels of government may at times conflict with one another.

This kind of situation can be frustrating when attempting to deliver services to clients. Furthermore, if the practitioner disagrees with a policy, he or she should attempt to change it. Lobbying for change of policies that have a negative effect on children in residential treatment is a professional obligation. It is critical for government at all levels to create policy that enhances the rights of children.

SUMMARY AND CONCLUSION

A brief history of the children's rights movement and the juvenile court system was offered in this chapter. It was emphasized that the juvenile justice system is much different from the adult criminal justice system. Residential treatment professionals must be sensitive to these differences.

It is also stressed in this chapter that residential treatment settings provide a great opportunity for practitioners to offer effective services to children and their families. Professionals working in residential treatment also must help to ensure that the rights of children in these settings are realized. Since children can be placed in residential treatment against their will, protecting their rights becomes an even greater professional obligation. Professionals working with children in residential settings must be familiar with the policies and procedures that help to ensure that the rights of children in this kind of treatment environment are not abused. Strategies outlined will prevent the abuse of children's rights.

The chapter also stresses that professionals working in residential treatment must cooperate with one another. If conflict does arise between professionals, strategies are offered that help to resolve this conflict. Finally, it was stressed in the chapter that professionals from various disciplines all contribute to successful treatment outcomes in residential settings. As services are delivered in this practice setting, it is critical for professionals to ensure that the rights of children are protected.

Chapter 6

Children's Rights and Protective Services

Protective services for children are available in every state. These agencies are designed to receive reports of child abuse and neglect from professionals and others. After receiving an allegation of child maltreatment, if warranted, protective services conducts an investigation. The primary focus of protective services is to identity services needed by families and children if an allegation of child maltreatment is substantiated.

When protective services provide intervention for families at risk, a service plan is outlined that includes the goals of intervention and the services the child and family need. This service plan must be approved by the court. A small percentage of children who have been abused and neglected are placed in foster care. More than 70 percent of the children in substantiated cases of maltreatment remain in their homes (Schere, 1991). This means that the services offered to families at risk must be effective. Schere (1991) concludes that the quality of these services varies greatly throughout the United States.

Since most children enter the protective services system because of child abuse and neglect, the chapter begins with a detailed discussion of the theory and research attempting to explain maltreatment of children. Some of these children must be separated from their parents; the psychological impact of separation and loss is therefore presented. The chapter concludes with the role and function of protective services in identifying and treating child abuse and neglect.

CHILD MALTREATMENT

Child abuse and neglect is a major social problem within the United States. For some time, there has been substantial interest in this problem. This interest has translated into numerous studies focusing on the causes and the identification of maltreatment. Scholars, practitioners, and policymakers continue to raise concerns about the quality of the research in this area. Many traditional notions about child maltreatment have been challenged by those seeking more enlightened explanations for why children are maltreated (Costin, Stoesz, and Karger, 1997).

Theory

Theories about child abuse and neglect have been slow to emerge; obviously, this lag in theory development has in turn hampered research as well as advances in practice. Much of the early theory in the field of child maltreatment concluded that the problem of child abuse and neglect was largely a personality disorder of the parents. The "battered child syndrome" identified by Kempe and colleagues (1962) is a classic example of the early theory building in the field. Kempe's early work essentially concluded that child maltreatment is an individual-based pathology and that the social environment plays a secondary role in its creation. Gladston (1965) argued a similar theme in the mid-1960s. To these theorists, child maltreatment is essentially caused by specific personality, behavioral, and emotional disorders. However, researchers such as Steele (1976) and Young (1964), using information provided by psychiatrists, psychologists, and social workers, refuted this perspective. Steele (1976) concluded that less than ten percent of parents who maltreat are seriously emotionally disturbed.

A great deal of the emerging theory is critical of the "individual pathology" approach to explaining child abuse and neglect. Current theory building is heavily grounded in the ecological perspective (Howze-Browne, 1988). An ecological perspective includes four factors for explaining human behavior. These are the individual, familial, social, and cultural factors.

Individual factors are characteristics that the parent and the child-victim possess as a result of their unique life histories and their physical and psychological attributes. The work of Garbarino (1977, 1991) goes into significant detail on these factors. The ecological approach, however, concludes that individual factors in and of themselves are not sufficient for explaining child abuse and neglect.

Familial factors are those that include the structure and function of the family system. Much of the theory on the familial structure has emerged from the field of sociology. Structural variables related to child maltreatment include but are not limited to single-parent families and families with a large number of children (Minuchin, 1967). Problems associated with family functioning include such characteristics as marital instability and family violence.

An ecological perspective also emphasizes social factors that include the quality of housing, presence of unemployment or underemployment, and formal and informal relationships. Oates (1989) and Hamilton (1989) in their work have identified numerous factors associated with the social context of child abuse and neglect.

Cultural factors are an intricate aspect of the ecological perspective. These factors include the all-embracing ideological fabric found within society. Some of the most important cultural values that have been found to be associated with child abuse and neglect are those that favor violence and corporal punishment. Vondra and Toth (1989) have attempted to illustrate in their work how cultural factors influence the problem of child abuse and neglect. Hamilton (1989) also argues that sexism and racism are critical factors related to child maltreatment.

The power of the ecological perspective is that it takes into account a confluence of variables, often identified by single-factor theories of child maltreatment, such as personality theory, and integrates these into a multifactor paradigm capable of being empirically tested (Pardeck, 1988). It should be noted, however, that the ecological perspective is far from the definitive explanation for child abuse and neglect. Even though the ecological perspective holds great promise, we still have a very limited understanding of the causes of child maltreatment. Even with this important limitation, a great deal more is now known about child abuse and neglect than just three decades ago. It is important that efforts continue at building sound theory in this area.

Unfortunately, child abuse and neglect is largely treated through individual counseling and other related therapeutic approaches, resulting in less than desirable treatment outcomes. The ecological perspective offers an alternative to individual-based interventions. However, the ecological approach cannot be implemented without fundamental changes in societal and professional values. As long as social policies within the United States continue to be grounded in the

belief that child abuse and neglect and other forms of family dys-
functions are simply a manifestation of individual aberration, an un-
supplemented individual treatment model will continue to be used.
This traditional model of intervention is grounded in the notion that
the core responsibility for rearing children is within the family system. Furthermore, the larger society is not obligated to provide social
and economic supports to families through policy efforts. Given this
dominant ideology found within the United States, child abuse and
neglect will remain a major social problem.

Research

Treatment interventions that appear to be most successful in treating child abuse and neglect are lay therapy, group parent education,
and self-help programs (Pardeck, 1989). Clients receiving long-term
treatment also appear to show increased positive change over those
who do not receive this kind of treatment (Pardeck, 1989). Even with
these important research gains, Costin, Stoesz, and Karger (1997)
conclude that human services personnel for the most part do not
know what is effective for dealing with the problem of child abuse
and neglect.

Much of the research on treatment outcome has been methodologi-
cally unsophisticated (Costin, Stoesz, and Karger, 1997). The variable that has been used in most research as a measure of successful
intervention is the reincidence of child abuse and neglect. A major
limitation of this variable is that not all subsequent incidents of abuse
and neglect are reported. Consequently, reincidence of abuse and neglect is only a rough measurement of treatment outcome (Kadushin
and Martin, 1988). Few studies in the area of child abuse and neglect
employ control groups.

Qualitative research focusing on child maltreatment is even less
precise than the empirical-based research (Costin, Stoesz and Karger,
1997). An example of the lack of rigor in the qualitative research is
reflected in the quote from Steele and Pollock's (1968) study focusing on the treatment outcome of sixty families:

> In the great majority of patients, treatment was successful,
> highly so in some, moderately so in others. Criteria of success
> were multiple. Of primary importance was a change in the style

of parent-child interaction to a degree which eliminated the danger of physical harm to the child and lessened the chance of serious emotional damage. (p. 138)

No details are reported in their research to support these findings. Similarly, Helfer (1975) concluded in his research that 70 to 75 percent of families at risk can be successfully treated with our present understanding of child abuse. The basis for Helfer's speculation was not presented in his research. These kinds of unsubstantiated conclusions continue to be indicative of much of the research in the area of child maltreatment (Costin, Stoesz, and Karger, 1997).

Finkelhor (1984) suggests that one of the most pressing research needs in the area of child abuse and neglect is to evaluate the effects of various treatment approaches. Communities throughout the United States are currently struggling with the development and implementation of programs aimed at treating child abuse and neglect. Oates (1989) concludes that future research needs to incorporate more sophisticated research designs, including control groups. Oates (1989) in his work has identified a number of rigorous studies that have implemented appropriate controls.

The current state of research in the field of child maltreatment is extremely limited. Research needs not only to implement comparison and control groups, but also to utilize more precise measurement tools. Howing and colleagues (1989) in their important work have identified a number of assessment tools now available to clinicians and researchers working in the field of child abuse and neglect. These assessment and research tools have been developed by researchers from a number of different disciplines. These tools assess individual, familial, and environmental functioning within an ecological context.

Milner (1986) developed the widely used *Child Abuse Potential Inventory* (CAP). This instrument measures child abuse at multiple levels, including individual, family, and environmental. Consequently, child abuse is viewed by Milner as a dynamic process that is ecological in scope and nature. Milner (1989) suggests that the CAP Inventory, among other possibilities, can be used as a screening tool for potentially abusive parents, as well as an instrument for evaluating program effectiveness, and as a general research tool. Milner (1989) argues, however, that the CAP Inventory must be used in a responsible fashion by not only clinicians but also researchers. This point should be noted for all clinical instruments.

Bavolek (1989) has developed the widely used Adult-Adolescent Parenting Inventory (AAPI) (available at http://www.aapionline.com). Like Milner's inventory, extensive research has gone into the development of the AAPI. Bavolek's inventory is based on the maltreatment theory that has developed over the years. Specifically, Bavolek developed the AAPI around four major factors often associated with child maltreatment: inappropriate developmental expectations, lack of empathy toward children's needs, belief in the use of corporal punishment, and reversing parent-child roles. Bavolek (1989) concludes that the AAPI can be useful in four important areas of assessment and research:

1. Assessing the parenting and child-rearing attitudes of adolescents and young adults prior to parenthood.
2. Assessing the parenting attitudes of parent populations for treatment and prevention purposes.
3. Screening potential foster parents, child care staff, and day care workers.
4. Examining the factors associated with abusive parenting that increases our knowledge of child maltreatment.

The research that has been conducted in the area of child abuse and neglect often lacks rigor and sophistication. Future research should make better use of the numerous research and assessment instruments now available. Using these research tools with improved controls will greatly enhance our understanding of the problem of child abuse and neglect.

Practice

Successfully treating child abuse and neglect is a very difficult task. Traditional psychodynamic approaches have been the core practice models for treating this serious social problem. One of the major limitations of these models is that few studies have found them to be effective. If one views the problem of child maltreatment from an ecological perspective, it becomes evident why such practice models do not work well with families at risk. Specifically, psychodynamic approaches do not consider such important factors as the client's family and the influences of social and cultural factors on the client's total social functioning. Schmitt and Beezley (1976) conclude that an alternative to psychodynamic approaches should include an ecological perspective. They suggest the following should be the core components in assessing and treating child maltreatment:

1. A comprehensive assessment of the child's family system and other systems affecting family functioning.
2. A multidisciplinary team approach for decision making and treatment intervention.
3. The use of diverse treatment approaches.
4. Periodic assessment of the intervention process.

Obviously psychodynamic treatment can be a part of these components; however, it is not the dominant treatment theme. The vital components stressed by Schmitt and Beezley are the family system and assessment that occurs throughout the treatment process.

The work of Pardeck (1989) and Wiehe (1989) is grounded in the treatment strategy advocated by Schmitt and Beezley. Both Wiehe and Pardeck have emphasized the role of the family system in successfully assessing and treating child maltreatment; they have also stressed the utility of the ecological perspective. The ecological perspective, given its dynamic orientation to treating child abuse and neglect, incorporates a multidisciplinary approach and emphasizes the importance of assessment of treatment outcome.

The ecological approach to practice suggests that behavior of individual family members can best be understood through the concept of *transaction*. What this concept means is that behavior of individual family members is shaped and molded through contact with other family members. Sameroff (1975) provides an excellent example of the transactional process:

> The mother who comes to label her infant as "difficult" may come to treat the child as difficult irrespective of his or her actual behavior. [T]he child . . . will come to accept "difficulty" as one of the central elements in his or her self-image, thereby indeed becoming the "difficult" child for all time. (p. 66)

The concept of transaction provides important insight into child maltreatment. The transactional process suggests that the practitioner should not presume that the child is a passive recipient of the abuse process; instead, the parent and child are partners in the process. However, the child is not a willing partner.

Wiehe (1989) has also noted that the therapist must be sensitive to the influences of the larger society on the family. It is important to consider the influence of sociocultural factors as a cause of child maltreatment. Narrow views do not adequately consider the role that sociocultural factors play in child abuse and neglect. Treatment approaches that do not consider these important variables often lack efficacy.

Family therapy appears to be one of the most effective approaches for treating child maltreatment because the practitioner can consider numerous factors, including the pressures flowing from the social environment. As pointed out by Pardeck (1989), reoccurring themes are found in many families at risk, including rigidity in interaction between family members and low levels of ego differentiation. Practitioners should carefully analyze these factors when assessing families at risk for child maltreatment. Therapists treating child maltreatment also must be sensitive to sociocultural issues influencing the family system, particularly the impact that poverty has on child abuse and neglect (Costin, Stoesz, and Karger, 1997). Families below the poverty level are often at great risk for child abuse and neglect. When considering child maltreatment from an ecological perspective, sociocultural variables such as poverty are extremely important factors to include in the assessment and treatment process (Costin, Stoesz, and Karger, 1997).

MALTREATMENT OF HOMELESS CHILDREN: AN ANALYSIS OF THE ADULT YEARS

Over the past two decades the number of homeless children has dramatically increased. Most of these children are members of low-income families and simply do not have access to housing. The author of this book has conducted a study on the number of homeless adults who experienced maltreatment as children. As the reader will observe, homelessness and child maltreatment are related variables.

Child maltreatment is clearly a major social problem leading to various impairments, both psychological and social. The extent of these effects varies depending on the child's age when maltreated, the severity and duration of the maltreatment, the type of maltreatment, and the personality makeup of the child. Maltreatment falls into three categories: physical, emotional, and sexual abuse. Each of these has a different impact on the child and may affect the child as he or she moves through the life cycle (Downs et al., 2004).

Physical abuse is the most common kind of child maltreatment. Physical abuse may result in the child being very aggressive or very withdrawn. The child may complain of soreness, wear inappropriate clothing to cover his or her body and may be afraid to go home or simply run away. As the child matures, inappropriate levels of aggression may be displayed when interacting with others. What is known from the research is that many individuals who end up in the penal system have a history of physical abuse (Downs et al., 2004).

Children vary in how they react to emotional abuse. Some children may direct their anger from being abused outward and become physically or verbally aggressive. Others will turn their pain inward and thus become at risk for suicide, drug and alcohol abuse, and depression. These kinds of problems have long-term consequences and may require treatment throughout the life cycle (Downs et al., 2004).

Evidence suggests the effects of sexual abuse can last into adulthood. Adults who were sexually abused may have sexual disturbance or dysfunction and have signs of diagnosable anxiety disorder and depression. Children who have been sexually abused are also more likely to experience revictimization that includes battering, sexual assault, or rape. Women with emotional disabilities also often have a history of sexual abuse (Downs et al., 2004).

What is very clear from the research is that physical, emotional, and sexual abuse has long-term consequences for individuals in terms of their social and emotional development. When children are abused it is critical for these victims to have appropriate treatment. A number of treatment modalities have been found to be effective in treating child abuse; these include individual counseling and family therapy intervention. Unfortunately, within the United States, many children who have been maltreated do not receive the appropriate treatment; this means the consequences of abuse become long-term and often last into adulthood (Pardeck, 2002).

Little research has been conducted on child maltreatment and homelessness; this is why the author conducted his study. Most of the studies have focused on the general problem of family violence and not specifically on the problem of child maltreatment. The research on family violence includes a study by Whitbeck and Hoyt (1999) who found that family violence is particularly high among homeless women and children. A 1990 Ford Foundation study found that 50 percent of homeless women and children were fleeing from abusive environments (Zorza, 2002). Thirteen of the twenty-nine cities surveyed by the U.S. Conference of Mayors identified family violence as a primary cause of homelessness (Waxman and Hinderliter, 1996). Finally, Pardeck and Rollinson (2002) found a high rate of violence among homeless women.

Method

The author's research analyzed case records of clients who received services from a large homeless shelter located in a predominantly rural region in the Midwestern United States. The exploration of the research topic included both quantitative and qualitative data.

Using a table of random numbers, 296 client files (20 percent of the sample population) were drawn from a 1999 roster of 1,480 homeless people entering the shelter studied. Forty-nine percent of the total sample of 296 homeless people were women; 82 percent of the sample was white. Fifty-five percent of the sample was twenty to thirty-nine years old; 33 percent was forty to sixty-four years old. Only two percent was over sixty-five. Fifty percent of the total sample had experienced some form of violence; 66 percent of the homeless women in the study had a history of violence.

Physical violence was the most common form of violence found among the homeless sample with emotional disabilities. Fifty-nine percent of the sample fell into this category. Of this group, 59 percent experienced physical violence during childhood, 14 percent during adulthood, and finally, 27 percent experienced physical violence during both childhood and adulthood. The next most common form of violence among the homeless sample with emotional disabilities was emotional abuse; this totaled 21 percent of the subjects. The majority of these (79 percent) experienced emotional abuse during childhood; 8 percent during adulthood, and 13 percent during childhood and adulthood. Thirteen percent of subjects experienced sexual abuse in their lives. As would be suspected, the vast majority, 90 percent, experienced sexual abuse during childhood. Five percent experienced sexual abuse during their adult lives and 5 percent during both child-hood and adulthood.

The author also explored themes of child maltreatment recorded in the case records of the homeless in the research sample. The following case narratives provide examples of the child maltreatment that the homeless experienced during childhood.

Father abusive: physically, sexually, and verbally

Violence with family of origin

Physical, sexual, verbal, and emotional abuse—family very dysfunctional

Sexual abuse by father

Emotional abuse by biological father; stepfather molested ages twelve to fourteen; physical and emotional abuse

Child's father physically abusive

Her stepfather physically and emotionally abused her

Father was physically and emotionally violent

Physically abused by her mother and first stepfather

Uncle molested her; father shot at her and stabbed her during early adolescence; mother was emotionally and physically abusive

Stepfather beat mother; violent neighborhood

Stepfather abusive

Adopted father very violent

Physical, emotional, and sexual abuse

Father is verbally abusive

Has experienced physical and sexual abuse

Stepfather abusive toward her

Aunt and uncle sexually, mentally, and emotionally abusive

Father was abusive physically and mentally

Stepfather physically and emotionally abusive; also, all of the males (brothers and uncles) were abusive

Physical, mental, and emotional abuse in foster care; her uncle sexually abused her repeatedly; abuse of every kind

Parents left child alone all day without supervision; emotional abuse and neglect

Stepmother beat her up

Sexually abused by family friend

Uncles physically abusive

Brother molested her between ages four and seven
Father of four of her children was very abusive
Father violent when drunk; wife murdered their two children

This research has illustrated a linkage between homeless adults and a history of child maltreatment. This is simply another example of the effects of poverty and other related social problems on children. As mentioned earlier in this book, one of the most serious attacks on children's rights is poverty. The findings in the author's study suggest that poverty places children at greater risk for homelessness and maltreatment.

SEPARATION AND LOSS

When children are placed in foster care and adoption they often experience separation and loss. The impact of separation and loss on children is age related. Younger children have a much different response to separation and loss than what older children experience. The treatment strategies offered by protective services build these differences into the services they offer. The following discussion covers issues related to the impact of separation and loss on children.

Behavior that children exhibit after placement in foster care and adoption is often predictable. Professionals can develop greater insight into the unique problems that foster and adoptive children experience through an increased understanding of the effect of separation and loss on human beings. The following offers problems often resulting from separation and loss. Many of these issues are common to children placed in foster care and adoption (Pardeck and Pardeck, 1998).

Everyone experiences separation and loss at various times of the life cycle. Without separation, it would be impossible for human beings to develop socially and emotionally, learn to make choices, and to mature. What is important for young children is to be able to separate from a parent for a short time period, for example, going to preschool, and to maintain a connectedness to parents when in care of others (Pardeck and Pardeck, 1998).

Bonding is the process that helps children deal with separation from parents. Bonding helps children carry a consistent internal picture and memory of the parent within the self; this process is referred to as object constancy. If this process is developing normally, separation from the parent, such as a child attending school, should go well. However, if separation experiences in childhood are problematic due to overindulged bonding and earlier failures to separate, the child may develop problems in childhood and later life. Ongoing issues throughout the developmental cycle of human beings is to maintain appropriate balance between attachment and self-actualization, between connectedness and identity establishment, and between dependence and independence (Pardeck and Pardeck, 1998).

When children experience separation and loss due to placement in foster care or other similar life events, they often react in predictable ways. These reactions may involve psychological pain and can even carry over into adulthood. Separation and loss is a core problem that children face in substitute care. For these children the separation experience is not just an event taking place at one moment in time, but instead is something they often must deal with into adulthood. When children separate from a significant other, such as a parent or other caregiver, the following are predictable responses (Pardeck and Pardeck, 1998).

When a child is confronted with a significant loss or separation from a caregiver because of placement in foster care, a predictable initial response is for the child to feel dazed. The child may wonder, "Why me?" The days following placement in care often have little meaning. It is also difficult for the child to concentrate and to feel good about himself or herself (Pardeck and Pardeck, 1998).

Loss due to separation from biological parents may also result in children having psychosomatic problems. These may include shallowness of breath, fatigue accompanied with the inability to sleep, and loss of appetite (Pardeck and Pardeck, 1998).

Children who experience significant separation from their biological parents sometimes go through a mourning process. An important stage of the mourning process is testing and accepting the reality of loss. Until the child realizes the separation is long-term and may be permanent, he or she will not be convinced of its finality (Pardeck and Pardeck, 1998).

Denial is the psychological process that keeps the hope alive that the parent(s) and child will be together again. In the child's mind, denial helps him or her to control and attempt to change events. The child feels if he or she wishes hard enough, the separation from his or her biological parent(s) can be undone. Once the child accepts the reality of being in placement, denial fades as the loss sets in; however, it may never completely disappear (Pardeck and Pardeck, 1998).

Anger is often a reaction to separation and loss. Given what has happened to a child, feelings of anger about being placed in care are understandable. Sometimes this anger is an attempt to redo the past, thereby attempting to change it. For example, a child in a foster care placement may do everything possible to get moved to a new placement; through this behavior the child repeats the abandonment trauma in hopes that this time he or she will emotionally master the separation and loss from his or her biological parents (Pardeck and Pardeck, 1998).

Anger may also be internalized and directed at the self; this may result in guilt. An example of this process is the child who blames himself or herself for being placed in an adoptive placement. If this sense of guilt about placement is not resolved, the child may continue to feel emotional pain (Pardeck and Pardeck, 1998).

Fantasies of a reunion with parents are particularly pronounced if a child feels a great deal of guilt. Even love can be a source of guilt for the child. For example, a child may resist accepting an adoptive family because doing so might show disloyalty to the absent biological parent. Hostility is often a reaction to a situation where a child is torn between conflicting loyalties (Pardeck and Pardeck, 1998).

Depression may result when anger is turned inward. An example of this process is the child who accepts the finality of an adoptive placement and therefore often experiences depression. Some children feel helpless and emotionally drained when depression begins to dominate their lives. It is difficult for children in such a circumstance to realize that they are not alone; if they continue to feel isolated and alone with their problems, the depression may increase (Pardeck and Pardeck, 1998).

Separation for some children is a source of embarrassment. Even though they know they have done nothing wrong and that they are not the cause of their placement in care, they still feel embarrassment. Feelings of embarrassment are particularly pronounced for children in placement when they attend school.

A typical reaction to separation and loss is fear. For example, the child placed in an adoptive home may fear that his or her new parents will decide to give the child up again, as his or her biological parents did earlier. Underlying the fear of many children who experience separation and loss is the question, "Who will take care of me if I don't live with my parents?" Professionals must work with children to help them deal with the fear that accompanies placement (Pardeck and Pardeck, 1998).

It is common for children to feel sadness along with the other predictable emotions that accompany separation and loss. Often children who experience loss feel unhappy for a while; over time these feelings are replaced with more positive feelings. To adults, this behavior makes little sense, but to the child it is a way of coping with separation and loss. The child becomes preoccupied with everyday living because the sadness is so great; if the child did otherwise, he or she would be overwhelmed by feelings of loss. Responding to sadness in such a fashion also allows the child to have some degree of control over the emotional pain that he or she is experiencing (Pardeck and Pardeck, 1998).

Children who do not immediately react to separation and loss may displace their feelings on other events. The foster child might, for example, displace his or her feelings about foster care when viewing a child on a television show who loses his or her family. If mourning of separation and loss is delayed or absent entirely, this condition at times suggests future problems for a child. Grief is important because it allows the child to express the emotional pain associated with loss. If not expressed, the child may exhibit the pain with academic failure or even delinquent behavior. If the child does not express the pain associated with separation and loss, it may well inhibit healthy social and emotional development (Pardeck and Pardeck, 1998).

Continuity of Relationships

Separation and loss disrupts the continuity of relationships that children have with significant adults, particularly parents. When children experience separation it affects their physical, emotional, intellectual, and moral growth. Growth and development are disrupted when upheavals and changes occur in a child's environment; these disruptions have consequences for children that are age related. Research by Goldstein, Freud, and Solnit (1973) offer the effects of separation and loss throughout the life cycle of children.

From birth to approximately eighteen months, any change in the routine of a child in this age group often results in food refusals, digestive upsets, sleeping problems, and crying. These reactions can even occur if a child's care is divided merely between a parent and another caregiver. They are obviously more pronounced for a child entering placement. Moving from the familiar to the unfamiliar for the child causes discomfort, distress, and delays in the child's orientation and adaptation to his or her environment (Goldstein, Freud, and Solnit, 1973).

When children experience separation and loss in the infancy to toddler stage of development, a number of predictable behaviors occur. Children's attachments at this stage are thoroughly upset by separation. For example, if a child is abandoned during this stage, the child will probably suffer from distress and anxiety. He or she may have problems forming human relationships. This is one reason why young children often resist bonding with adoptive placement. If children experience a great deal of instability during the infancy to toddler stage of development, their emotional attachments become increasingly shallow and indiscriminate (Goldstein, Freud, and Solnit, 1973).

Preschool children who experience separation and loss may have problems bonding with adults. Children in this stage have a tendency to regress when they experience a lack of continuity of care. They may experience regression in their social and emotional development and lose their ability to communicate effectively with others (Goldstein, Freud, and Solnit, 1973).

School-aged children experiencing a lack of continuity of care may have problems with identification. When separation occurs during this stage, the attachment to and identification with a future caregiver becomes increasingly difficult. For example, the foster child who is moved frequently during the school-aged stage may cease to identify with any set of substitute parents. Children who have been placed in care may develop negative attitudes toward their biological parents. These attitudes may also result in the new caretakers becoming scapegoats for the shortcomings of the biological parents. These kinds of attitudes and behaviors may result in dissocial or antisocial behavior (Goldstein, Freud, and Solnit, 1973).

The adolescent child in placement may project the aura that he or she is not affected by the separation and loss from the biological family; however, this impression is often misleading because it is simply a coping mechanism. Independence for adolescent children is extremely important because it helps them develop their individual identities. Challenging authority figures is also a normal behavior for adolescents; however, for a successful outcome in identity development, the breaks and disruptions of attachment should come exclusively from the adolescent child (Goldstein, Freud, and Solnit, 1973).

Adults who as children experienced disruptions in their lives may treat their children as they themselves were treated. This behavior may continue a cycle costly for the next generation (Goldstein, Freud, and Solnit, 1973).

PROTECTIVE SERVICES

Protective services are specialized services aimed at treating neglected, abused, exploited, or rejected children (Kadushin and Martin, 1988). The focus of protective services is preventive and nonpunitive and is geared toward rehabilitation through identification and treatment functions which underlie the need for intervention. The following quote from the work of Kadushin and Martin (1988) defines protective services:

> [Protective services is] based on law and is supported by community standards. Its purpose is protection of children through strengthening the home or, failing that, making plans for their care and custody through the courts. . . . [It is] a service on behalf of children undertaken by an agency upon receipt of information which indicates that parental responsibility toward those children is not being effectively met. (p. 218)

The need for protective services arises when parents do not provide appropriate care for their children. The legal doctrine of *parens patriae* provides the legal sanction for protective services to help families that may be at risk. Under this doctrine, the state has an obligation, as a "parent" to all children, to defend the rights of children. With the doctrine of *parens patriae,* a third party is introduced into the parent-child relationship; this provides children with some assurance of outside protection and support (Kadushin and Martin, 1988).

The Process of Protective Services

The protective services intervention process can be viewed as consisting of the following stages. These stages are adapted from the work of Kadushin and Martin (1988):

1. Prevention
2. Investigation and the social history
3. Assessment
4. Planning
5. Treatment
6. Evaluation
7. Case termination

Each of these stages is viewed in sequence. All are part of the services delivered by protective services agencies throughout the United States.

Prevention

Preventing problems before they occur makes sense to most practitioners. The three kinds of prevention are primary, secondary, and tertiary. Primary prevention anticipates family problems and prevents them from occurring. Secondary prevention provides prompt relief to families confronted with problems. Tertiary prevention offers rehabilitative efforts to reduce the residual effects of a problem. This kind of prevention typically occurs only after the family problem is well established within the family system.

The ideal kind of prevention is obviously primary. Few treatment programs are of this nature. If the child welfare system stressed primary prevention, the need for protective services would be greatly minimized. Protective services typically offer secondary and tertiary prevention. More often than not, tertiary prevention has been the norm for service delivery because the problems within many of the families who enter the protective services system are well entrenched.

Investigation and the Social History

The legal reporting of suspected child maltreatment triggers this stage. Laws require that mandated reporters, such as social workers and teachers, report suspected abuse and neglect. Professionals have been held liable for failing to do so (Kadushin and Martin, 1988).

Upon receiving a complaint of suspected child maltreatment, protective services must decide to conduct an investigation. If the complaint appears to have merit, the agency must act in a timely fashion. Investigation often begins with a check of any previously recorded protective services data. An investigation must be done in a timely manner before bruises or welts disappear.

During the investigation, protective services attempts to balance the rights of children against those of the parents. The preliminary investigation is designed to ensure that the child is safe and to ascertain the needs of the family. A complete social history of the family is also conducted; this is extremely important information for determining the presence of abuse or neglect. At no time is the identity of the complainant disclosed. Once the investigation is completed, a decision is made concerning the need for protective services.

Assessment

Assessment of child abuse and neglect is extremely difficult. As noted earlier in this chapter, it is difficult to identify families at risk. The causes of child abuse and neglect have been difficult to identify. The theory development in this area has also been weak.

Bavolek (1989) has noted four dominant themes in abusive families. These include parents who have inappropriate developmental expectations of their children, parents who lack empathy toward their children, parents who have strong beliefs in corporal punishment, and parents who reverse roles with their children. Even though these factors are far from being sound predictors of child abuse, they certainly have been found to be associated with abusive families.

It has been extremely difficult to identify traits of parents who abuse their children versus those who are neglectful. It has been suggested that practitioners should use different assessment tools for those two kinds of child maltreatment because they have little in common (Kadushin and Martin, 1988).

The protective services practitioner must largely rely on practice experience when assessing for abuse and neglect. It is very difficult to develop a typical profile for parents who maltreat their children.

Planning

Once an assessment is made for protective services, a case or permanent plan must be developed. When developing a plan it must be assumed that parents have the ability to change. Practitioners must be sensitive to the fact that often the child's parents are the only ones the child has known. Even though children may have been abused or neglected by their parents, children of families who maltreat have often bonded with their parents. The plan should be guided by the following philosophy:

1. The birth families have the capacity to change and provide appropriate care for their children.
2. It is the child welfare system's role to work collaboratively with the families when developing a case or permanent plan.
3. Plans are designed to assure continuity in a child's life.
4. Services are time-limited, with measurable outcomes.
5. The plan is designed to provide for the safety of the child and to help parents meet their children's needs.
6. If the child is in substitute care, the caregivers must be part of the planning process. One of the practitioner's roles is to problem solve with the caregivers to help them fulfill their role of caregiver for the child.

Chapter 1 presents a thorough discussion of why the case or permanent plan must have the following elements. Goldstein, Freud, and Solnit (1973) provided the philosophical grounding to the permanent plan in their book, *Beyond the Best Interests of the Child.*

Treatment

When a report of alleged child maltreatment is substantiated, protective services must provide help to the family. As would be suspected from the earlier discussion in this chapter, casework counseling is the most common form of treatment provided (Kadushin and Martin, 1988). Most maltreated children remain in their own homes (Schere, 1991); approximately 20 percent are placed in foster care (Kadushin and Martin, 1988). Protective services may offer day care services, homemaker services, and other related forms of support and intervention.

It is important for the practitioner to establish rapport with the family at risk. A core objective of treatment is to attempt to ensure that parents will call the agency for help if there is a crisis (Kadushin and Martin, 1988).

Evaluation

Evaluation of treatment intervention by protective services should continue throughout the intervention process. The case or permanent plan is written with specific goals and objectives that are measurable; these allow the practitioner to make a reasonable estimate of the success of the intervention. As noted in this chapter, numerous assessment instruments are available to practitioners. These instruments can enhance not only the evaluation process but also can be used for research purposes.

Termination

A target date for termination is built into the case plan. The protective services agency makes the decisions for termination, not the parents. Before termination occurs, protective services must be sure the child will be safe. After termination, the agency may continue to contact the family at various intervals to ensure that the child is safe and his or her needs are being met.

THE COURT AND PROTECTIVE SERVICES

The juvenile court is greatly different from the criminal court. Criminal court attempts to establish guilt or innocence; the juvenile court is concerned with protecting children and prescribing treatment, not guilt or innocence. The goal of the juvenile court is to protect children who are not able to protect themselves. The juvenile judge should ideally be like a wise, affectionate, and caring parent.

Three types of children may enter the juvenile court system. These include children who are in need of supervision, delinquent children, and children who have been abused and neglected. The following discussion focuses on children who have been maltreated.

All states have legislation describing under what conditions the juvenile court can intervene into the parent-child relationship. These laws differ from state to state; however, the following is the typical process used in cases of child abuse and neglect throughout the United States.

The process begins with the *petition.* The petition is a request for the court to make a decision about a child who has been brought to the attention of the protective services agency. A decision must be made at this time to either allow the child to remain in his or her home or to be placed in substitute care on a temporary basis. A temporary placement can last up to three days.

The *jurisdictional hearing* is the next phase. During this phase the judge decides if the evidence collected by protective services is sufficient to sustain an allegation of child abuse or neglect. If the evidence does not substantiate child maltreatment, the case is dismissed. If the evidence is present, the case is continued to the *dispositional stage.*

The core goal of the dispositional stage is to decide if the child should remain with his or her parents or be placed in substitute care. Alternatives for placement include placement with a relative, placement in foster care, or placement in a residential setting. At the dispositional stage, the following issues are addressed:

1. Visitation by parents if the child is placed in substitute care.
2. The development of a case or permanent plan.
3. The next date for the court to review custody of the child.
4. Who is to pay for the child's maintenance—this is typically the state's responsibility.
5. Payment of the court-appointed attorney's fees, including the guardian ad litem and the parent's attorney if court appointed.
6. The projected date for jurisdiction of the child's care to cease.

The case plan that is developed outlines the goals and objectives of treatment for the child and the family. This plan is reviewed from time to time to help ensure its success. Once the goals and objectives of the treatment plan are achieved, the juvenile court no longer has jurisdiction over the child. The juvenile judge has great latitude in deciding what happens to children who enter the juvenile justice system. As stressed in Chapter 2, the judge must decide the "best interest" of the child. Not only is this standard vague, but so are the child abuse and neglect laws found in various states. This means child advocacy is often called for by practitioners and others in order for the child's rights to be protected in the juvenile justice system.

Providing Testimony to the Court

Child advocates and others working with children in the juvenile justice court system should follow a number of rules when giving testimony in court. The following outline provides strategies for giving effective testimony and special concerns for cross examination.

Guidelines for Giving Effective Testimony

1. Be prepared. Preparation is the key to effective testimony.
2. Answer only the question asked. Do not volunteer information. "Rambling" answers are not permitted in court. The opposing attorney would not have the opportunity to object to certain types of inadmissible evidence if he or she did not know the general area of information to which you were about to testify. The opposing attorney may not be able to discern this general area from the questions asked; thus you are required to limit responses to only the information asked of you.
3. If you do not understand the question, ask that it be repeated. If you still do not understand, say so. Never guess at what a question means.
4. If you do not know the answer to a question, say so. Never guess. This is particularly important for your credibility. If the opposing attorney and/or the judge discovers that you are guessing at the answer, no matter how insignificant the information seems, other answers you have given may also appear as guesses. Many times, your credibility will be strengthened if you admit when you do not know answers to certain questions.
5. If you are asked a yes-or-no question and feel that such an answer is misleading without an explanation, state that you cannot answer the question properly with a yes or no, but that the answer requires an explanation. You have a legal right to explain.

6. Be exact in your testimony. For example, say "one p.m." instead of "around noon," or "nine visits" instead of "numerous visits."
7. Take time in answering questions. Think before you answer. Do not be hurried by the attorney who is questioning you.
8. Show respect for the court. Dress conservatively. Be prepared and knowledgeable about the case.
9. Be as objective as possible. Try to avoid taking sides. Your role is to present evidence to the court, not to win the case. Appear confident about your abilities and your factual observations; do not appear nervous or defensive.
10. Unless specifically asked for your opinion, limit your testimony to your factual observations.

Special Concerns of Cross-Examination

Cross-examination is often the most difficult part of testifying. The attorney may attempt to discredit the practitioner's testimony, particularly if it has been damaging to his or her client. Discrediting or impeaching a witness is part of the adversary process of the court system. It is important to remain calm during cross-examination. Do not become angry or defensive with the attorney. This is easier to do if you understand the purposes of cross-examination and that such questioning is not to be taken personally.

It is also important to understand and anticipate some of the strategies commonly used by the attorney during cross-examination. These strategies include:

1. Pointing out discrepancies between the social worker's report and testimony in court, or between statements in direct examination and statements in cross-examination.
2. Showing that the practitioner dislikes the parents and is therefore biased against them.
3. Showing that the practitioner did not provide any real support to the family.
4. Showing that the practitioner is inexperienced.
5. Demanding that the practitioner answer with a yes or no, when questions cannot be adequately so answered.

6. Showing that the practitioner made prior, out-of-court statements that are inconsistent with the practitioner's statements in court.
7. Question the accuracy of the observation or memory of the practitioner.

In addition, attorneys frequently attempt to intimidate a witness with a disrespectful attitude, abrasive tone, repetitious questioning, sarcasm, or indications of disbelief. These attempts to anger or rattle the witness into making a careless or discrediting statement are generally the most difficult part of cross-examination.

SUMMARY AND CONCLUSION

This chapter outlines the role of protective services for children who may be at risk for abuse and neglect. If maltreatment is substantiated, protective services is mandated by law to provide services and treatment to children and their parents. The identification of families likely to maltreat children is difficult. The research literature provides very few rigorous studies that have identified the causes of child abuse and neglect. It also reports that few distinctions have been found between families at risk for maltreatment and those who are not. Given this situation, protective services has a very difficult legal mandate to fulfill.

The chapter also provides an in-depth study on the relationship between homelessness and child maltreatment. The study concluded that when children experience maltreatment it increases the probability that they may experience homelessness, not only as children but also as adults.

The following points are critical to child advocates working with protective services (Schere, 1991):

1. All legitimate reports of child abuse and neglect must be investigated and assessed.
2. All children needing protection from abuse and neglect where parents or caregivers are unwilling or unable to provide care to their children should receive services.

3. Adequate services must be provided to strengthen families and to prevent future maltreatment; these services should be provided in the child's home whenever safety permits.
4. When services do not prevent placement in substitute care, a safe, stable foster home needs to be identified along with a plan for family reunification and parental visitation. Within a reasonable time frame, family reunification should be attempted.
5. When it is not possible for children to be safe in their own homes, a permanent plan should be developed for adoption; long-term, stable foster care; or some other form of placement.

According to the Child Welfare and Adoption Assistance Act of 1980 these points are mandated by law. At times, advocacy is called for in order to ensure that a child's rights are being protected under the law in the protective services system.

Chapter 7

Advocacy and Children's Rights

The goals of advocacy include achieving social justice, empowering people, and creating positive social change. Advocacy helps individuals correct situations that are unjust. Achieving social justice through advocacy requires the active participation of people who are vulnerable or disenfranchised; advocacy clearly is an important strategy for improving the well-being of children. The banding together of those who wish to achieve social justice provides the opportunity for empowerment for active, responsible participation in public affairs (Lewis, 1992). The role of the advocate is to speak on behalf of individuals and to empower them to speak on their own behalf in those situations where their rights have been denied. The advocacy role is a critical strategy for enhancing children's rights because it brings children's issues to the public's attention. Laws and legislation are often only enacted after the public perceives issues as unjust (Pardeck, 1996).

McGowan (1987) argues that advocacy can be conducted at two levels, case advocacy and cause advocacy. The case advocacy approach focuses on individual cases, such as a single child whose rights have been violated. It involves the advocate's intervention on behalf of a client or identified client group with one or more secondary institutions to secure or enhance needed services, resources, or entitlements (McGowan, 1987). Cause advocacy seeks to redress collective issues through social change, such as creating or improving social policies. An example of this might be advocating for child and family policies at the state and national levels.

Rees (1991) argues that case and cause advocacy both begin by identifying the dynamics causing the injustice. Rees concludes:

> The decision to pursue the advocacy of a case or a cause, or a combination of both, will usually have been preceded by the

identification of an injustice which it is felt cannot be rectified simply by efficient administration or negotiation. The identification of an injustice and the sense of conviction that the removal of this injustice should become a priority. . . . It is not sufficient merely to recognize an injustice. You have to believe that this issue should be fought for, and if necessary over a long period of time. (p. 146)

The effective advocacy role involves data collection, effective communication with the public through the media, raising revenues, building coalitions, and other related strategies.

Miley, O'Melia, and DuBois (1995) suggest the following points should be an integral part of the advocacy process:

1. The location of the problem creating the social injustice must be identified. It must be determined if the problem reflects a personal need, a gap in services, or inequitable social policy.
2. The objectives of advocacy must be identified. Objectives might be defined as procuring entitlements for children or expanding job opportunities for parents.
3. The target system of an advocacy effort must be identified. At times this system might be the advocate's own agency or other systems the agency works with.
4. The advocate must determine what authority he or she has to intervene in a targeted system. This can include legal rights of children and judicial decisions related to children's rights.
5. The resources supporting the advocacy efforts must be identified. These resources include professional expertise, political influence, and one's credibility in the community.
6. It must be determined the degree to which the target system is receptive to the proposed advocacy effort. The target system will make this decision based on the reasonableness or lawfulness of the advocacy intervention.
7. The level at which the advocacy will occur must be analyzed to ensure that the desired outcomes will be achieved. Different levels of intervention might include policy changes, modification of administrative procedures, and alterations in the discretionary actions taken by staff of a human service agency, school, or other related organizational setting.

8. The object of the advocacy effort must be identified. This might include individual service delivery, agency administrators, a legislative body, or other similar social systems.
9. The strategies of advocacy intervention must be determined. These strategies include the roles of negotiator, collaborator, and adversary.

Those involved in advocacy efforts must learn and grow from the outcomes of prior advocacy efforts, including both failures and successes. What is also important to remember is that advocacy is a process that includes skill, timing, and planning. Furthermore, advocacy is a holistic approach to social change that involves efforts at the micro-, mezzo-, and macrolevels (Pardeck, 1996).

Those who are involved in advocacy efforts must understand when to use this strategy as a means for achieving social justice (Pardeck, 1996). If one considers, for example, the rights of children with disabilities, advocates need to be aware that many public and private entities may not agree with the laws protecting special needs children. Many systems located in the public and private sectors, including public schools and private businesses, would prefer self-regulation over federal mandates aimed at protecting children with disabilities. However, self-regulation does not necessarily work and even with the passage of legislation, such as IDEA and the ADA, social systems mandated to conform to disability laws will attempt to avoid compliance. This means advocacy is an absolute necessity to help ensure disability laws are implemented appropriately (Pardeck, 1996).

Entities legally bound by the mandates of civil rights laws such as the ADA attempt to avoid compliance for a number of reasons. First, organizations, including public and private schools and private businesses, have been provided the compliance materials for the ADA; however, they often do not comply because the law may contradict bureaucratic rules of these systems. For example, the child with a disability brings a unique set of needs to the school, including the need at times for reasonable academic accommodations. Schools are often rigid social systems and are not prone to make exceptions; they literally must be forced to make exceptions through strong advocacy efforts (Pardeck, 1996).

Second, all public and private entities bound by the mandates of laws such as the ADA argue that they operate on limited resources. If the parent of a child with a disability requests a reasonable academic accommodation in order for the child to attend school, the school may perceive the request as nothing more than an added cost. Advocates must play the role of convincing schools that compliance with laws such as the ADA is mandatory and that reasonable academic accommodations for persons with disabilities under the ADA is based on the needs of the person with a disability and not necessarily the needs of the organization's budget (Pardeck, 1996).

Third, individuals are often intimidated by both public and private bureaucracies. Bureaucratic structures have a tendency to reinforce this intimidation. For example, a parent of a child with a disability may have limited experience and exposure in dealing with the organizational structure of a school. The parent may need the help of an advocate in dealing with this structure. Skillful advocates understand how complex organizations work and are well aware of the regulations these systems must follow by law and administrative regulations (Pardeck, 1996).

Last, often it is difficult for the person with a disability or the parents of a child with a disability to look at issues objectively. Skillful advocates are able to step back from situations that negatively impact their children and bring objectivity to the advocacy process (Pardeck, 1996).

Advocates understand that even though laws and legislation are enacted, they are not necessarily implemented. Advocacy is about making sure organizations follow the rules and regulations that they are mandated to implement. Advocates realize at times they must use power and influence to force organizations to comply with the law (Pardeck, 1996).

APPROACHES TO ADVOCACY

The following provides a brief overview of the various approaches to advocacy (VeneKlasen and Miller, 2001). Each of these approaches can be used to help ensure that children have their rights realized. Advocates for children need to identify the system that is preventing a child or a class of children from having their rights met and then apply the approach or approaches that will be most successful in overcoming the problems created by that system. Advocates may use multiple approaches of advocacy aimed at a system that has created barriers to children's rights. For example, a state social service system may have an unreasonable policy that prevents low-income children from qualifying for Medicaid; in order to change this policy advocates may use two approaches to advocacy—protest and litigation. That is, child advocates may wish to bring the unreasonable Medicaid policy to the attention of the news media through public protest. They may also aim litigation toward forcing the state social service system to make it easier for low-income children to qualify for Medicaid. Each of the following approaches to advocacy has been used successfully in the children's rights movement.

Collaboration

This approach to advocacy is used when there is compatibility and agreement between grassroots organizations advocating for children's rights and government. This collaboration with government is designed to implement legislation or needed services for children. Similarly, government may give joint grassroots organizations the task to monitor the legislation or needed services to help ensure they are properly implemented.

Protest

A demonstration or march relies on numbers and creative messages to gain attention and support of the public. A march of 2,000 people will not usually have the impact of one with 35,000 people. Timing is critical. Boycotts are another form of protest often directed at systems preventing children's rights. Vigils are a less confrontational expression of protest. Protest is sometimes a tactic of last resort, used when more conventional approaches of influence have failed to open up a policy dialogue.

Litigation

Litigation has been an extremely powerful approach used very successfully in the children's rights movement. A well-publicized court case can draw public attention to a problem and lead to legal reform that helps children. A class-action lawsuit can be a very powerful tool for helping a large number of children who have had their rights denied. One advocacy group, Children's Rights, has been very successful in using this form of advocacy. Some examples of their work are given later in this chapter.

Public Education and Media

Education and media strategies build public support and may influence policymakers involved in children's rights issues. Strategies include providing data, articles, and alternative policies to the media, as well as creative messages using music and videos. Alternative media strategies using theater, posters, and pamphlets are especially useful in areas where media outlets are limited.

Research

Position papers and proposals based on solid research increase the credibility of advocacy. Research provides the necessary information for planning, policy alternatives, and lobbying. Depending on the methodology used, research can also strengthen alliances, build constituencies, and help develop citizenship skills. Where information is hard to get, research efforts can evolve into "right to know" advocacy strategies. Advocacy usually benefits from close ties with sympathetic researchers and policy analysts who give child advocates speedy access to facts and analysis in the midst of political battles.

Persuasion

Advocacy efforts must be persuasive to a wide range of audiences. Persuasion has three main ingredients:

1. *Lobbying* involves attempts to meet face-to-face with decision makers to persuade them to support a children's rights issue or proposal.
2. *Clout* is gained through the credibility and legitimacy of demands; by showing strength through mobilizing popular support for children's rights; by working in coalitions and with many diverse allies; and by using the media to inform, educate, and be visible.
3. *Negotiation* involves bargaining to seek common ground or, minimally, respect for disagreement in the area of children's

rights. It happens between allies, advocates, and constituents as well as across the table with those who have power. To bargain with decision makers, advocates need to know their power and their opponent's, as well as what is negotiable, what is not, and what needs to be done if negotiations fall apart.

Organization and Constituency-Building

The long-term nature of most advocacy efforts aimed at children's rights demands strong links with constituency groups. Effective advocacy requires alliances between organizations and with key individuals for leverage, legitimacy, and implementation of children's policy. Organization for children's rights depends on effective decision making, shared leadership, clear roles, communication, and members and staff with analytical skills and confidence.

Empowerment

A vital component of all advocacy efforts aimed at children's rights is empowerment. Empowerment is geared toward strengthening people's confidence and understanding of power. People's awareness of themselves as protagonists with rights and the responsibility to participate in and transform political processes is the core of active citizenship concerned with the well-being of children.

EFFECTIVE ADVOCACY SKILLS
FOR PARENTS

This section offers effective advocacy skills for parents by focusing on the rights of children with disabilities. These skills can also be used by parents when they advocate for the rights of their children in other kinds of situations. What is emphasized is that parents must be patient and skilled in the advocacy process in order to be effective.

IDEA, the ADA, and other disability laws have been enacted to protect the rights of children with disabilities (Pardeck, 1998). Parents have a primary responsibility for ensuring that their special needs children receive appropriate services as mandated by law. Parents often have the greatest knowledge about their children's disability and needs, both medical and academic. They must be sure that their child's rights are being realized in the school system. This can be achieved if parents learn how to effectively advocate for their special needs children. The following strategies and skills are designed to help parents become more effective advocates. The goals of the following are to empower parents and to ultimately achieve social justice for their special needs children in the school system.

Parents Must Believe in Their Rights

Parents must be taught that they are equal partners with other professionals in the school system that work with their children. Equal partnership also means that parents must accept their share of responsibility for solving problems and in making plans for their children's services.

Parents Must Have a Clear Vision

Parents must learn to communicate clearly with school officials, including teachers. They must be realistic and optimistic about what they can achieve. In other words, while trying to achieve what is perceived as ideal, they must be able to recognize what is realistic.

Organization

Parents must be taught to understand that being organized is a necessity to effective advocacy. Parents must know how to file information and keep track of records and other important documentation needed for the future. Parents must realize that it is difficult to be an equal partner with school officials if they do not have the same information as the school. Parents should be encouraged to date all materials and to make duplicate copies of all documents.

Prioritize

Parents must develop skills in learning how to decide what the most important issues are related to their special needs children. This should be based on the needs of their children. One useful technique is to list these needs on paper and then prioritize each need in order of importance. Needs should be stated in positive terms; this makes them less threatening when presented to school officials.

Understanding Children's Disabilities

Parents of a special needs child must learn everything possible about their child's disability. It is important to acquire in-depth information about the medical needs of their child, as well as the various assistive technology needed by them. In general, parents often know more about the needs of their children than professionals. It is important for parents of special needs children to share information with school officials and to draw upon the expertise of various professionals involved in the schooling of their children.

Parents Must Know the Laws

Parents must learn about their rights for their children under IDEA, the ADA, and other disability laws. It is also useful to become familiar with their rights under FERPA (Federal Educational Rights and Privacy Act). By knowing these laws, they will be better advocates for their children.

Parents Must Follow the Chain of Command

It is important for parents to know that effective advocacy means they should first start with the classroom teacher before going to higher authorities when advocating for their children. Teachers should be allowed the opportunity to address issues before parents as advocates move to higher levels of the organizational structure. If results cannot be obtained first with a teacher, then parents must move systematically up the chain of command.

Parents Should Be Informative

Parents of special needs children should learn how to help teachers understand the needs of their children. These include what motivates their children, their likes and dislikes, and the teaching approaches that have worked in the past. Parents should make a special effort to convey all relevant information to the school officials in order to enhance their child's learning experience.

Parents Should Offer Solutions

Parents need to be creative in finding solutions to problems confronting their special needs children. Positive solutions are those that benefit everyone involved in the lives of their children. Since teachers and other staff cannot be experts on all disabilities, it is important for parents to share their knowledge with professional staff. This important information can be very helpful for finding solutions to problems confronting special needs children.

Parents Must Be Principled and Persistent

It is important for parents to master the art of being clear to school officials concerning their children's needs and to stand firm with their position on these needs. It is important for parents to keep at the advocacy process and not to let the battle become the issue. Parents must avoid being adversarial and realize that they must be assertive and not aggressive. Parents must have a vision that issues will be resolved to their satisfaction. It is best to assume that school officials, including teachers, have honorable intentions.

Parents Must Learn to Communicate Effectively

Parents must understand that many issues result from poor communication between them and the school. Parents of special needs children must learn to listen to what others are saying and to realize that others may have valuable insights into a problem confronting them. If parents do not understand something, they must ask questions. Parents must be sincere and honest, and say what they really mean. Effective communication involves smiling, being relaxed, and not making others defensive. It is a good idea for parents to follow up conversations and meetings with a written summary of the discussion and agreements made.

Parents Must Let Others Know When They Are Pleased

Parents of special needs children may take things for granted until there is a problem. It is important for parents to realize that they should express satisfaction and excitement when their children are succeeding; school officials appreciate this kind of feedback. Everyone appreciates compliments for doing a good job.

Parents Must Develop Endurance

One of the first lessons one learns from doing advocacy is that it is important to have endurance. Advocacy is a process that takes time. Parents of children with disabilities will face many challenges and issues; some successes and some failures must be expected. It is important to learn from these experiences. Parents must realize they will be working with school districts for many years to ensure that their child's educational needs are being met. Effective advocacy skills and efforts will help make this relationship a positive one.

Parents Must Follow Through

Parents of special needs children must make a concerted effort to monitor the progress of their child's education. It is important that parents make sure that the goals and objectives agreed to for their child's education are being realized. Parents of special needs children can always renegotiate the educational program for their children if they feel it is necessary to do so.

Parents Must Have a Sense of Humor

Advocacy takes time and is largely about endurance. Developing and cultivating a sense of humor is one of the most important traits for parents to develop if they are to be successful advocates.

LITIGATION AND CHILD ADVOCACY

Children's Rights (2004), a national advocacy organization, uses its expertise to build the political and public pressure needed to compel child welfare bureaucracies to change. Children's Rights puts failing systems under close scrutiny, identifies problems, and generates solutions. When a system fails to respond, Children's Rights brings litigation to force reform and then monitors implementation to ensure that children's lives actually get better.

For over thirty years, Children's Rights has been a leader in creating new law and obtaining sweeping court-ordered decrees that serve as a model for reforming child welfare systems nationally. Originally a project of the American Civil Liberties Union, Children's Rights became an independent nonprofit organization in 1995.

The Goal of Children's Rights

Children's Rights' (2004) goal is to ensure that the child welfare system follows the laws affecting children's lives. These laws deal with the following areas:

1. Laws that keep children safe from abuse and neglect.
2. Laws that are aimed at children receiving adequate medical, mental health, and educational services.
3. Laws that help to ensure that children are returned to their families whenever possible or, through the adoption process, helped to find a permanent, loving family.

Challenges of Children's Rights

The following identifies the challenges of the Children's Rights (2004) national advocacy organization. These are challenges for all child advocates:

1. Over 3 million children in the United States are reported victims of abuse and neglect each year.
2. There are 600,000 abused and neglected children currently placed in foster care.
3. Foster care should be safe and temporary. However, children stay an average of three years. One hundred thousand languish over five years—reabused, neglected, or denied education and health care they desperately need to thrive.

Action Agenda of Children's Rights

Children's Rights (2004) creates meaningful change in dangerous child welfare systems through advocacy, policy analysis, public education, and targeted litigation. The action agenda for Children's Rights includes the following:

1. Expose what happens to children in failing child welfare systems.
2. Educate the public on why specific systems fail and how they can be fixed.
3. Create programs and initiatives to prevent abuse and neglect and benefit endangered children.
4. Utilize the power of the courts to compel government systems to fulfill their legal mandates on behalf of children.
5. Interact with child welfare advocates, professionals, and policymakers to share insights and advance a common agenda.

Examples of Successful Litigation by Children's Rights

The following reviews examples of successful litigation by Children's Rights (2004). These cases have been litigated over the past several decades.

Juan F. v. Rell: *Connecticut*

When Children's Rights first became involved with this case, Connecticut's underfunded and overburdened Department of Children and Families (DCF) routinely put children at risk of harm. DCF failed to provide appropriate placements and basic services for foster children and failed to adequately investigate reports of abuse and neglect. Social workers carried caseloads twice the national average. Training for workers was grossly inadequate and DCF lacked the ability to track basic data and information on children in state custody. The lawsuit, filed in 1989, resulted in a comprehensive consent decree in 1991. Since then, Children's Rights has been working with a court-appointed monitor to watch over DCF's performance. Children's Rights has addressed noncompliance through negotiations and, when necessary, through court proceedings to enforce the consent decree.

Although considerable improvements have been made in areas such as overall funding for DCF, the creation of a comprehensive training program and an information system that can accurately track critical information concerning children, the state and DCF have repeatedly failed to comply with numerous areas of the consent decree.

In February 2002, the court approved an eighteen-month transition plan, which shifted emphasis from the specific "process" requirements of the consent decree to a more flexible management system, under which DCF agreed to meet specific outcome measures. If DCF met the measures, and if they could sustain their success, the plan would have allowed the state and DCF to exit from the consent decree and court involvement. In the summer of 2003, the monitor released several reports which concluded that DCF had failed to meet court-ordered goals in most of the fundamental areas, found that DCF was routinely depriving foster children of opportunities to be adopted, and found that, rather than improving children's lives, "multiple traumas associated with long lengths of stay in DCF custody, such as multiple placements, separations from siblings, abuse in custody, and multiple social workers, worsened their emotional and mental health" (*Juan F. v. Rell,* H-89-859, http://www.childrensrights.org/Legal/Juan_Rowland.htm).

As a result of this dismal performance, and in light of over a decade of the state's making and breaking promises to its children, on October 7, 2003, Children's Rights obtained an extraordinary court order approving a new agreement reached between the governor and DCF commissioner that avoided a contempt hearing and possible court-ordered receivership. Under the new agreement, the state admitted its longstanding noncompliance and failures. For the first time ever in the nation, management authority over the state foster care system has been transferred to the federal court through the court monitor, with the consent and cooperation of the governor and DCF commissioner. The agreement created a three-member task force that included the monitor, the senior state budget official, and the DCF commissioner, with ultimate power over the department in the hands of the federal court. On December 23, 2003, the monitor released his exit plan, the blueprint that will govern the department's performance for the next three years. The exit plan contains twenty-two concrete measures in fundamental areas of child safety, permanency, and well-being. If DCF can meet these measures by November 2006, federal court oversight will end; if DCF fails to comply, oversight will continue until the improvements are made. Under this new agreement, the federal monitor has the powerful potential to bypass political and bureaucratic barriers that have prevented change for so many years. Unfortunately, in January 2004, the state challenged a straightforward provision requiring them to provide the resources necessary to implement the exit plan. Plaintiffs opposed and the court strongly rejected the state's maneuver. With this political setback behind us, plaintiffs are hopeful that the new agreement will allow for the kind of sweeping changes in management and accountability—and, most important, improvements in the lives of abused and neglected children—that have been lacking in Connecticut for so long. Children's Rights will continue to be a watchdog over the state's compliance with the new agreement.

LaShawn A. v. Williams: *District of Columbia*

Staggering caseloads, lack of services, overcrowded foster homes, and almost no adoptions were all evidence of the failures plaguing the DC child welfare system, which was then part of the Department of Human Services (DHS), when Children's Rights became involved in reforming the system. Once children entered the foster care system, they were unlikely to leave until they were old enough to be on their own.

In June 1989, Children's Rights initiated a massive reform effort by filing a class-action suit in federal court alleging DHS's failure to comply with the federal Adoption Assistance and Child Welfare Act, the U.S. Constitution, and various local statutes. In 1991, after a full trial on the issues, in which Children's Rights presented overwhelming proof that the district had harmed children in its custody, District Court Judge Thomas Hogan issued a 102-page opinion declaring his "inescapable conclusion" that DHS had violated the plaintiff children's rights. Unfortunately, DHS made only minimal progress between 1991 and 1995, prompting the court to impose the drastic remedy of a receivership on DHS. That decision marked the first time in history that a child welfare system was placed under full receivership by a court because of its noncompliance with court-ordered reforms. In 2000 the new administration of Mayor Anthony Williams expressed that the district would change and be committed to reform if it regained control of the system. Among other plans, the district expressed commitment to form a new, cabinet-level Child and Family Services Agency (CFSA).

In light of these commitments, the court terminated receivership in 2001 and put the district on probation. The probation period ended in January 2003. Children's Rights and the court monitor will continue to watch CFSA's progress very carefully to ensure that the current administration stays on its course of progress.

Bonnie L. v. Bush: *Florida*

The state of Florida has over 15,000 foster children, and its Department of Children and Families (DCF) has no place for many of them. By 2000, approximately 20 percent of Florida's foster homes were operating over their licensed capacity and, as a result, children removed from their families were often placed for long periods in overcrowded, "temporary" holding facilities without necessary treatment. DCF was also known to rent motel rooms to serve as housing for foster children.

In August 2000, Children's Rights joined local Florida advocates in a lawsuit against DCF. Before the case made it to trial, however, the district court dismissed most of the plaintiffs' claims, accepting DCF's contention that the suit might interfere with the operations of Florida's dependency court—a "state's rights" argument typically rejected by federal courts in these cases. On the claims not dismissed, the plaintiffs reached a settlement whereby DCF agreed to reinforce a nondiscriminatory policy toward African Americans and older children who are about to "age out" of the system. The plaintiffs also appealed the dismissal decision. In May 2003, the Eleventh Circuit Court of Appeals affirmed the district court's dismissal, holding that each individual foster child within the plaintiff class may seek relief from the harms they are suffering only through their separate dependency court cases despite the fact that the dependency courts are precluded as a matter of law from granting the systemic relief foster children in Florida so desperately need. After unsuccessfully seeking to have the Eleventh Circuit reconsider its decision, plaintiffs filed a petition with the U.S. Supreme Court seeking review of the Eleventh Circuit's gross expansion of the so-called "abstention" doctrine, which has the result of closing the federal courthouse doors to

Florida's foster children. By order dated November 3, 2003, the Supreme Court denied this petition, effectively ending the case.

Despite legal roadblocks faced thus far, Children's Rights and its Florida allies have called national attention to Florida's ailing child welfare system. Children's Rights also succeeded in pressuring DCF to emphasize nondiscriminatory policies and to respect the privacy of plaintiffs' medical records. Though the *Bonnie L.* litigation is now over, Children's Rights is considering other types of legal action, including state court litigation and differently focused federal court litigation aimed at protecting Florida's foster children.

Kenny A. v. Perdue: *Fulton and DeKalb Counties, Georgia*

On June 6, 2002, Children's Rights filed this suit, charging that Georgia's Department of Family and Children Services (DFCS) in Fulton and DeKalb Counties is overburdened and mismanaged, placing children at high risk. The lawsuit challenges a system that is failing the very children it is supposed to protect. Among many systemic problems, children are placed wherever a bed or a slot is open and not according to their needs. Social workers have crushingly high caseloads that prevent them from monitoring the safety of children in foster care. Children face further abuse and neglect at an alarmingly high rate while in state custody.

In addition, when the case was filed, Children's Rights found children languishing for months in dangerous emergency shelters without needed services. In the shelters, foster children of all ages were living in dirty, overcrowded conditions and exposed to violence, sexual assault, prostitution, gang activity, and illicit drug activity. Because the shelter conditions were so grave, the plaintiffs filed for a preliminary injunction, demanding that the DeKalb and Fulton shelters be closed immediately. Ultimately, an injunction was not necessary because DFCS promised to close the shelters. In fact, both shelters were closed by February 13, 2003. The court found that "few concrete steps were taken to close the shelters before this lawsuit was filed."

Since then, the heart of Children's Rights' reform lawsuit has continued to move forward. In August 2003 Children's Rights won a significant ruling from the court, which granted class-action status and ordered that the case proceed to trial on behalf of all 3,000 foster children in Fulton and DeKalb Counties concerning violations of their federal and state rights while in foster care. In September 2003, in the wake of several recent child deaths, both the commissioner of the Georgia Department of Human Resources and the director of the state Division of Family and Children Services resigned. However, the dangerous failures plaguing DFCS will require fundamental changes to the system itself, not a mere rearrangement of leadership. Children's Rights continues the fact-finding discovery process in the lawsuit, collecting information to prepare for trial. Children's Rights and their cocounsel at the firm of Bondurant Mixson & Elmore in Atlanta have reviewed over 100,000 pages of documents and have taken the deposition testimony of over thirty state and county child welfare administrators and managers. Factual discovery has been completed and expert reports have been exchanged. Efforts for a mediated settlement are currently underway.

Olivia Y. v. Barbour: *Mississippi*

A federal civil rights lawsuit was filed on March 30, 2004, in the U.S. District Court for the Southern District of Mississippi charging that the Mississippi Division of Family and Children's Services (DFCS) has placed thousands of children under its care in danger and at risk of harm and has left many thousands more to fend for themselves in abusive and neglectful homes. The lawsuit, *Olivia Y. v. Barbour,* seeks to stop ongoing violations of children's rights and to ensure that DFCS adequately cares for and protects the state's children.

Olivia Y. v. Barbour was filed on behalf of six named plaintiffs—children who have suffered physical and psychological harm while in DFCS custody or who have been simply abandoned by DFCS. The class action case is also brought on behalf of the nearly 3,000 foster children who are currently dependent on DFCS for their care and protection, as well as the thousands more who are improperly diverted from the system. The lawsuit asserts that for more than a decade, the state has been well aware of its pervasive failure to serve the children who depend on DFCS for their basic safety and most fundamental needs and has failed to provide the leadership, support, and resources necessary to protect and care for these children.

G. L. v. Stangler: *Kansas City, Missouri*

In 1977, Legal Aid of Western Missouri filed suit against the state of Missouri because of grave inadequacies within Kansas City's (Jackson County's) foster care system. Children's Rights was asked to join the suit soon thereafter. In 1983, the parties entered a settlement as a legally enforceable, court-ordered consent decree. In 1985, the court ordered the creation of an independent monitor. Despite these actions, significant reforms came about only after a 1992 contempt finding after full trial on the issue of noncompliance, which jeopardized the state commissioner's job and forced him to address the foster care system's severe underperformance.

A national panel of experts was convened after the contempt trial to review the foster care system and issue recommendations. In 1994, the panel recommended specific ways to speed reform, and these suggestions were incorporated into a new consent decree and exit plan that was negotiated by the parties and entered by the court as a new order. Since 1994, with intensive efforts from both parties to solve problems rather than litigate, the Division of Family Services (DFS) has come into compliance with many major elements of the consent decree. For example, DFS has achieved commendable compliance in areas such as case planning, service provision, certification/licensing procedures, and health care planning. Acknowledging these successes, the parties entered a revised consent decree and exit plan in 2001, and allowed DFS to exit the components of the previous consent decree for which goals had been achieved.

Charlie and Nadine H. v. Codey: *New Jersey*

In New Jersey, slashed funding and years of official neglect resulted in a child welfare system so deficient that a blue ribbon panel, created by the governor in 1997, compiled a list of almost 400 recommendations for reform. The state responded with a defective strategic plan, which barely scratched the surface of problems, and a funding increase that failed to reinstate former funding levels. Moreover, the state flatly refused Children's Rights' offer to work with the Division of Youth and Family Services (DYFS) to better the system.

This lawsuit was filed in August 1999 after it was clear much-needed reform would not occur without the pressure of a lawsuit. In

June 2003, after the death of Faheem Williams, a child well-known to DYFS who was found beaten to death in a Newark basement along with two starving siblings, and after the plaintiffs compiled massive evidence of the state's egregious failures, the parties reached a landmark, legally enforceable settlement agreement. The agreement stipulates areas of immediate and long-term action. For example, the state must begin by allocating $23.85 million in funding for new DYFS employees, space, equipment, and foster homes. DYFS will also conduct an immediate safety assessment on children presently in DYFS custody and move children from unsafe homes and facilities. The state will immediately allocate $1.5 million just to recruit new foster homes for these children. The agreement requires DYFS to work closely with a panel of independent experts to create a reform plan. The panel will specifically set the legally enforceable outcomes that DYFS must achieve. The panel may disapprove DYFS's plan, in which instance the case returns to court with liability stipulated by the state and the only issue for trial will be what remedy should be imposed. After an eighteen-month period of oversight, the panel will dissolve and an independent monitor will take its place. The district court approved the settlement agreement at a hearing on September 2, 2003, and entered it as a court order stating:

> it is clear that this settlement, indeed, is fair, appropriate and probably, if anything, long overdue. I think it represents the best that can be presented in the U.S. legal system and represents the highest ideals and achievements of attorneys who, when the time is right, can put aside the adversarial process of our legal system and achieve the result which, in fact, will better society and, in particular in this case, achieve hopefully long overdue reforms in our child welfare system.

Children's Rights will remain actively involved to ensure DYFS's compliance with the settlement agreement.

On February 18, 2004, Governor James McGreevey submitted a 188-page reform plan for approval by the panel. Key elements include adding over 1000 casework staff positions, capping caseloads, increasing reimbursements to foster parents, developing more housing and substance abuse services for families, reducing multiple placement moves for foster children, and moving children more quickly into permanent homes. The plan commits to budgeting for

DYFS an additional $125 million in the first year and $180 million in the second year, representing an increase of over 30 percent in overall DYFS funding. The expert child welfare panel has submitted to the court a first monitoring report, analyzing the state's accomplishments and shortcomings thus far. Should no agreement be reached on the required reforms, the federal district court can ultimately set the requirements for reform.

Joseph and Josephine A. v. Bolson: *New Mexico*

In 1980, Children's Rights and local attorneys filed this suit against officials of what is now known as New Mexico's Children, Youth and Families Department (CYFD). CYFD was making virtually no effort to place children, many of whom suffered abuse and neglect, with permanent families. The parties settled in 1983 and entered a consent decree. Initially, CYFD made some progress, but reforms stalled.

In February 1998, after years of litigation about the state's noncompliance with the consent decree, the parties entered into a court-ordered "stipulated exit plan" (SEP), which specified benchmarks that must be met before the court terminates supervision over CYFD. Despite this new agreement, CYFD continued functioning at unsatisfactory levels. A 1999 review of case plans indicated, for example, that only 29.6 percent of children's cases had an appropriate, current treatment plan reviewed every six months. In October 1999 the plaintiffs filed a new contempt motion regarding CYFD's noncompliance with court-ordered standards. The state responded by filing a motion to dismiss the entire case using an arcane legal argument. Agreeing with the state's position, the district court dismissed the entire case. However, Children's Rights appealed and in January 2002 the Tenth Circuit Court of Appeals reversed the dismissal and remanded the case for further proceedings.

On January 16, 2003, in a sweeping legal victory, the district court reaffirmed the enforceability of the SEP. On September 27, 2003, Children's Rights and its cocounsel signed a memorandum of understanding with CYFD officials intended to focus CYFD's efforts at fixing the problem that has plagued New Mexico's child welfare system for decades: finding permanent families for children whose goal is adoption.

On November 26, 2003, the new agreement was signed as a federal court order to replace the current court-ordered SEP. The innovative agreement calls for CYFD to hire two expert consultants to create adoption resource teams (ARTs). These teams will meet with CYFD caseworkers on every case where a child's permanency goal is adoption in order to create an individualized adoption plan (IAP) that will identify each child's specific barriers to adoption and set forth steps to break down those barriers. CYFD will be bound to carry out these steps, and the teams will meet on each case every sixty days until the children have permanent homes. Compliance with the new agreement will be monitored by a neutral third party.

Marisol v. Pataki: *New York*

The 1995 discovery of five-year-old Marisol locked in a closet and the death of six-year-old Elisa Izquierdo threw the media spotlight on one of the most expensive and dysfunctional child welfare systems in the nation. Children's Rights had been working for several years to bring the system's abuses to light, and in December 1995 filed a lawsuit on behalf of over 100,000 children subjected to the failings of both the New York State Office of Children and Family Services (OCFS) and New York City's Administration for Children Services (ACS).

In 1999, the parties reached historic settlements. The settlement with the city created an advisory panel of child welfare experts to help turn ACS around. This arrangement has produced substantial reforms in ACS. For example, ACS has achieved lower caseloads, obtained funding for additional placements, sharply increased staff training, vastly improved its data management system, and reconfigured foster care services along neighborhood lines. The settlement with the state required OCFS to implement a statewide child welfare data management system and to exercise oversight responsibility toward ACS, to evaluate ACS's handling of child fatalities, and to oversee corrective actions when fatality reports reflect ongoing problems.

The city settlement agreement expired in 2001, with substantial achievements having been gained. The state settlement agreement is still in effect as to the state's computer information system. Children's Rights went to court in 2001, for the state's failure to make sufficient progress in implementing the system, and is receiving semiannual reports from the state that detail the current status of implementation. Children's Rights will continue to monitor the state's progress in complying with the terms of this component of the agreement and will go back to court if necessary.

Brian A. v. Sundquist: *Tennessee*

For years in Tennessee, the Department of Children's Services (DCS) routinely housed children in emergency shelters and other temporary holding facilities for upwards of six months because the state had nowhere else to put them. Children in the system were also bounced through many inappropriate foster placements and, though the children stayed in state custody for extended periods, DCS made little effort to provide them with an education, return them to their parents, or arrange for adoption.

In response to requests from local advocates to investigate DCS's systemic failings, Children's Rights partnered with attorneys across the state in May 2000 to file a suit on behalf of the over 9,000 children then in DCS custody. Intense negotiations produced a settlement agreement in August 2001. The agreement, which is fully enforceable in court, imposes sweeping reforms on Tennessee's child welfare system. Since the August 2001 settlement, Children's Rights has been actively monitoring DCS's compliance with the terms of the *Brian A.* settlement, including numerous regular meetings with the independent monitor, representatives from the Tennessee Attorney General's Office, and numerous senior DCS administrators. Some needed reforms have been implemented. DCS has created, for the first time, a quality assurance division to ensure that children are being adequately served. DCS also hired 350 new caseworkers; closed an unsafe 250-bed orphanage-style facility; and closed numerous inappropriate "in-house" schools while increasing efforts to integrate foster children into public schools.

Notwithstanding these improvements, in November 2003, after reviewing the monitor's reports detailing DCS's failures to comply with most of the settlement's provisions, Children's Rights filed a motion in federal court asking Judge Todd Campbell to find state officials in contempt of court and to order immediate compliance with the terms of the settlement. The motion also asked the court to appoint an independent special administrator with the authority to develop and implement a plan to ensure Tennessee makes the many specific reforms called for by the settlement or, in the alternative, for an order requiring DCS to itself develop and implement such a plan.

On December 29, 2003, plaintiffs reached a stipulation with the state resolving the contempt motion. The stipulation, which has been approved by the court, requires DCS to work with a technical assistance committee (TAC) composed of five national child welfare experts to develop and put into effect a comprehensive and detailed "implementation plan." The plan, which is to be approved by the TAC and the court, is to be a blueprint for carrying out the many reforms called for in the settlement. It must address a number of identified problem areas for DCS by setting forth, for each substantive area, goals, strategies, action steps, benchmarks, persons responsible, and necessary and committed resources. The key terms of the implementation plan will be enforceable as a court order.

In the stipulation, the defendants concede that they have not fulfilled a number of terms of the settlement agreement. The stipulation also delays by fifteen months, from March 2006 to June 2007, the first date on which the defendants may seek to exit from any portion of the settlement agreement. To provide the defendants with breathing room to develop and put a suitable plan into effect, the plaintiffs have agreed not to seek a finding of contempt based on noncompliance with the settlement agreement for a period of twelve months, reserving the right to return to the court for any violation of the settlement agreement that endangers the safety or well-being of class members and to seek a finding of noncompliance/contempt for the defendants' failure to adhere to the central terms of the implementation plan.

Jeanine B. v. Thompson: *Milwaukee, Wisconsin*

It was well documented that Milwaukee County ran one of the worst child welfare systems in the country. Social workers' caseloads were deplorably high, necessary child services were unavailable, few children were being adopted, and the rate of neglect and abuse soared. Local advocates and experts requested assistance from Children's Rights and, in 1993, Children's Rights filed suit.

Responding to the pending litigation, the state took over the previously county-run child welfare system. However, when the state failed to deliver promised reforms, Children's Rights filed a supplemental complaint against the state. Finally, the parties reached a settlement and, in December 2002, the court approved a settlement agreement that sets performance targets for the Bureau of Milwaukee Child Welfare. The state is issuing public reports every six months on its progress in reaching the stipulated goals. Since Children's Rights became involved with the Milwaukee system, the system has improved in numerous ways. For example, caseloads that previously exceeded 100 children per social worker have dropped to an average of less than twenty-five children per social worker.

FAMILY POLICY AND CHILD ADVOCACY

The family system is the most important social institution to children. Parents perform a number of critical roles for children within the family system. These include (Westman, 1991):

1. Parents provide sustenance by ensuring that children receive food, shelter, and clothing.
2. They provide a critical developmental function for children through affectionate and restraining caregiving and parental modeling of coping skills.
3. Parents offer advocacy to their children through planning for, making decisions about, and negotiating children's sustenance and developmental needs in the community by arranging for housing, day care, health care, education, and social and recreational activities.

Parents vary, obviously, in their abilities to fulfill these critical parenting roles. What makes parenting difficult in the United States is the lack of a comprehensive, coordinated set of policies and programs aimed at supporting parenting efforts. The United States is the only developed country lacking these kinds of policies. The following offers an analysis of why this situation exists. The lack of a comprehensive family policy in the United States means child advocacy becomes even more important because so many children and family needs go unmet.

Barriers to Family Policy

Pardeck (1990), Rice (1977), and Schorr (1968) have identified several factors that appear to prevent the development of a national family policy in the United States. These include:

1. The tradition of emphasizing the individual over the family system.
2. A preference for minimal government intervention into family life.
3. The pluralistic nature of American society, which prevents agreement on the policies and programs needed by families.

The tradition in the United States is for minimal government intervention into family life. The public is concerned that such intervention would be counterproductive to family well-being. This tradition is grounded in the U.S. Constitution, which is silent on the subject of the family. The implied contract in the Constitution is between the individual and state—this has resulted in a vacuum in the area of family policy and programs.

The pluralistic nature of American society has made it difficult to reach a consensus on the role of government in family life. Pluralism has also made it difficult to define what is meant by the term "family." Until these kinds of barriers are overcome, a comprehensive family policy will not emerge (Pardeck, 1990).

Europe and Family Policy

The United States and Europe have much in common in the area of cultural traditions; however, they part on those traditions concerning family policy (Pardeck, 1990). Tropman (1985) offers an explanation for why Europe and the United States differ so dramatically in the area of children and family policy. He argues that Europe and the United States have unique religious traditions that help to explain why Europe has a highly developed family policy and the United States does not. Tropman (1985) claims that a dominant ideology that he labels the "catholic ethic" is the grounding for explaining why Europe has made great policy gains aimed at supporting families. The catholic ethic finds its roots in the Roman Catholic, Anglican, and Lutheran religious traditions. The United States is dominated by a very different religious tradition, the "Calvinistic ethic." This ethic emphasizes the importance of the individual and self-initiative. These two religious traditions create normative and value standards that are very different in four major areas (Pardeck, 1999):

1. Attitudes toward social problems,
2. Attitudes toward work,
3. Attitudes toward charity, and
4. Attitudes toward the welfare state.

Social Problems

The Calvinistic ethic views poverty as being caused by laziness and lack of motivation. This tradition divides the poor into worthy and unworthy categories. The worthy are seen as those who are not responsible for being poor, such as persons with disabilities who are poor. The unworthy poor are those who are seen as able to work, but who refuse to do so. The Calvinistic tradition highly values means tests and "safety nets" that are temporary solutions until individuals can find work. The recent welfare reform, the Personal Responsibility and Work Opportunity Reconciliation Act of 1996 is a classic example of a program based on the Calvinistic ethic. Calvinism also endorses a residual approach to policy development that tends to emphasize cost cutting over individual needs and is typically driven by crisis within American society (Pardeck, 1999).

The European catholic ethic presents a much different view of needy individuals and families. This ethic has been translated into programs grounded in the view that families have limited control over social problems and are often victims of them. Tropman (1985) suggests that the catholic ethic views excessive wealth as spiritually dangerous. Thus the distribution of wealth to families in need is seen as a citizen's duty. Consequently, an impulse toward mutual obligation and social welfare is the result (Pardeck, 1999).

The catholic and Calvinistic ethics help to explain why Europe and the United States differ in the area of family policy. All European countries offer some form of income supports for families; no such program exists in the United States. European countries offer health care to all families; approximately 40 million persons in the United States have no health insurance (Pardeck, 1999). The tax systems in

Europe tend to be progressive; they are regressive in the United States. European countries are largely composed of middle-class families and poverty is nearly nonexistent, whereas in the United States millions of families live below the poverty level. The Calvinistic ethic endorses the tradition of not supporting family programs; this has resulted in many American families going without critical social services, adequate nutrition, shelter, and health care (Pardeck, 1999).

Work

Personal worth is measured by individual productivity under the Calvinistic ethic. The catholic ethic suggests a much different view that emphasizes the worth of individuals based on what they contribute to society; thus work has an instrumental meaning reflected in providing clothing, food, and shelter for oneself and one's family. Under the catholic ethic, work is seen as a creative process that benefits the community and enhances the talents of individuals.

The Calvinistic ethic has influenced the worldview of many Americans toward the meaning of work. Work defines the very essence of how one perceives the self and others; those who lack work are seen as unworthy of social and economic supports from society. The Calvinistic ethic suggests that welfare programs stifle the work ethic. If anything these programs are seen as deterrents to work. Furthermore, a number of social theorists conclude that the true function of welfare programs in the United States is to regulate the poor (Piven and Cloward, 1971). Piven and Cloward argue that private industry has a vested interest in keeping welfare benefits low during times of economic prosperity to ensure an adequate workforce. A major argument against family allowances and other economic and social supports has been that such programs encourage relief over work (Pardeck, 1999).

European countries have a much different view of work; one that suggests the American orientation toward work is less than accurate. Even though Europe has highly developed family policies and programs, little evidence suggests that these policies stifle the work ethic (Pardeck, 1999). One might even argue that the inability of the United States to respond to the needs of children and families through policy and programs is creating a dangerous social class that might potentially destabilize the larger society. Presently, several million families are homeless in the United States; this is a major social problem that must be resolved (Pardeck, 1999). Postindustrial society demands that families receive adequate economic and social supports in order to stabilize the larger society. Health care, day care, and other family supports are a necessity in a postindustrial American society (Pardeck, 1999).

Charity

Tropman (1985) concludes that the catholic ethic stresses horizontal relationships between the individual and society, while the Calvinistic ethic offers a vertical view of social relationships. These views translate into different perspectives concerning the meaning of community (Pardeck, 1999).

Tropman (1985) suggests that the catholic ethic results in a greater sense of community and commitment to one another. This ethic may help explain why European countries have progressive tax systems that have created a large middle class and virtually eliminated poverty. It also provides insight into why most European countries have children and family programs. Such supports help the larger society realize its commitment to children. These kinds of programs illustrate commitment to the importance of horizontal relationships among community members grounded in the catholic ethic (Pardeck, 1999).

Calvinism takes a much different view than the catholic ethic concerning the meaning and importance of charity. Calvinism views charity as a negative that should be provided only under the most unusual circumstances. With such a worldview, it makes perfect sense that poverty, homelessness, and other social problems are far more common in the United States than Europe. Until this worldview changes, millions of children and families will not have their basic needs met within the United States (Pardeck, 1999).

Organizational Structure

The final aspect of the catholic versus the Calvinistic ethic concerns how each culture views the bureaucratic structures that deliver social welfare programs. The catholic ethic endorses the need for a bureaucratic structure as critical to effective social service delivery. Tropman (1985) argues that this tradition is connected to tolerance of a highly developed church structure that has simply been replaced by a developed welfare state. The Calvinistic ethic, as would be expected, has a much different position on the organizational structures critical to the delivery of social services. The Calvinistic ethic is suspicious of highly developed church structures; this view carries over to a strong distrust of a highly developed welfare organizational structure. Under the Calvinistic ethic, parents are responsible for most needs of their children, not the larger society (Pardeck, 1999).

The origins of the catholic and Calvinistic ethics are clear. The Calvinist reformation radically reduced or eliminated the medieval ecclesiastical institutional structure. Church policy became congregational; the pastor stood alone at the head of the local church assembly. That aloneness may well have given rise to the ideal of self-reliance, not merely in the religious sphere but in all aspects of life. The ideology of self-reliance has become a dominant theme throughout the United States and suggests that this ethic has resulted in underdeveloped children and family policies (Pardeck, 1999). Given this situation, child advocacy becomes a necessity to help ensure that children receive the basic needs of life including shelter, health care, and other important social services. Professionals play an important role in helping to ensure that children receive basic services and that their rights are realized through the advocacy process.

PROFESSIONALS AND CHILD ADVOCACY

Child advocacy in the United States is an extension of parental advocacy based upon the traditions of *parens patriae* and in loco parentis doctrines, both of which lodge responsibility for children with the state when parents cannot meet the needs of their children (Westman, 1991). The protective doctrine of *parens patriae* means the state has a general duty to protect all citizens, especially those incapable of protecting themselves, such as children. The doctrine of in loco parentis means an agent other than parents, for example the courts, can make decisions ordinarily within the province of parents. Professionals play a critical role in the implementation of the doctrines of *parens patriae* and in loco parentis.

Professionals, according to Westman (1991), have a resistance to conducting advocacy on behalf of children. For example, health workers have a tendency to be preoccupied with the treatment of disease, lawyers with legal procedures, educators with the mechanism of teaching, and social workers with administrative policies and paperwork (Westman, 1991). However, professionals have an obligation to correct those situations that are antithetical to the well-being of children. The following are techniques for conducting case child advocacy, a process that professionals have an ethical obligation to be involved in. These techniques are based on the work of Westman (1991). The techniques include the following:

1. *Fact finding*—A technique that is designed to identify families at risk.
2. *System linking*—This technique involves the coordination of child welfare service.
3. *Needs determination*—The goal of this technique is to determine the capacity of parents to meet the needs of children.
4. *Child involvement*—This technique is designed to help ensure that children are involved in the advocacy process.
5. *Developing objectives*—Objectives aimed at support, strengthening, or replacing parental sustenance are involved in this technique.
6. *Resolving conflict*—When conflict arises between individuals in the child welfare and other systems, the use of this technique becomes critical.
7. *Implementing a plan*—Children who are at risk need a life plan; the goal of this technique is to accomplish this task.
8. *Protecting children's rights*—This technique is designed to ensure that the legal rights of children are protected in the court system.

Fact Finding

This technique involves sensitivity to the emotional and developmental needs of children in the family system. These needs are identified through conducting an assessment of the parent-child relationship. This assessment will indicate if protective services or other similar kinds of supports and treatment are needed. Disturbed parent-child relationships are typically caused by abuse and neglect, alcohol and drugs, and emotional disabilities.

System Linking

The linking of professionals and the services they provide are a critical part of the advocacy process. For example, professional advocacy involves the input of teachers, social workers, and other professionals when families are at risk. This technique includes planning conferences that are designed to include information from a variety of professional perspectives about the needs of children they are working with. This interpersonal context is important among professionals because a child may act much different with one professional versus another. These different perspectives on the child will offer a more accurate assessment of the child's needs.

Needs Determination

A third technique is determining a child's sustenance, developmental, and advocacy needs and the capacities for families to meet these. Information for making these determinations can be drawn from schools, the courts, and other professionals who are familiar with the child and his or her family. Since advocacy is a drastic process, superficial assumptions about a child or family are inappropriate. Specific information about a particular family system is essential to effective child advocacy.

Child Involvement

The fourth technique is involving the child in the advocacy process. For example, children often do not understand why they are being placed in foster care or adoption. Professionals must interpret to children what is happening to them. If children have the cognitive and emotional developmental capacity, this technique involves soliciting input from children, focusing on how they perceive their own needs. At minimum, this technique demands that the professional must establish rapport with children who are in need of advocacy efforts.

Developing Objectives

This fifth technique involves the development of objectives that will guide the advocacy process. Objectives depend on the extent to which families can care for children and the needs of their children.

Objectives include the resources that parents may need to care for their children. They might include the procurement of services for children, such as counseling. They may include objectives aimed at strengthening parenting capacities through therapy, training and education, in-home services, or other early intervention approaches for helping families at risk.

Resolving Conflict

This important technique is almost always a critical aspect of successful advocacy. It is nearly impossible to avoid conflict when the rights of parents and children clash. Conflict also often occurs between children, parents, schools, neighborhoods, and other systems. Successful advocates are able to resolve or minimize the negative effects of conflict.

Implementing a Plan

An example of this advocacy technique is the permanency plan required for all children placed in foster care. This plan often extends over time and involves an interdisciplinary advocacy team, parents, and children if they are old enough. The permanency plan must be flexible and designed to adapt to the changing needs of children.

Protecting Children's Rights

The eighth technique is protecting the rights of children. Child advocacy often creates an important tension between the rights of children and their parents. It is critical that the advocate ensures that children have legal counsel, due process, and equal protection under the law. The guardian ad litem and Court Appointed Special Advocate (CASA) volunteer are examples of individuals who use this technique for protecting the legal rights of children.

A CASE EXAMPLE: GARY

This is the case of Gary, a special needs child who has been placed in foster care (Pardeck, 1988). The case covers efforts made by a guardian ad litem assigned to Gary's case. The case is presented and then analyzed in terms of the previously presented professional advocacy techniques.

Gary, a two-year-old boy, was underdeveloped both physically and intellectually. The child's vocabulary consisted of approximately three words and he was not able to walk more than two steps without assistance. The child was diagnosed as having fetal alcohol syndrome. Gary's parents were both alcoholics and unemployed when Gary was placed in foster care. The family was not receiving any kind of public assistance.

The guardian ad litem assigned to Gary's case had his first opportunity to interview Gary's family during a two-hour home visit with his parents while a number of relatives were also present. The guardian ad litem observed the interaction patterns between Gary and the family.

During the home visit, the guardian ad litem began the assessment process of Gary's family system. He concluded that Gary's parents did not interact with him in a typical fashion. The mother in particular held the child for no more than two minutes during the home visit; the father did not interact with the child at all. When the child was not playing on the floor, he was passed from one relative to the next. The mother commented several times during the home visit about how curious Gary had always been about "things" in his environment and how active the child was. These comments were totally out of touch with the child's physical and intellectual behavior.

One week after the visit, the guardian ad litem did an extensive interview with each of the parents and one of the relatives present at the home visit a week earlier. Gathering this information helped to assess the needs of Gary and the intervention needed to help Gary return to his biological family. Through the interview, the guardian ad litem learned that both parents continued to abuse alcohol; this was confirmed by Gary's parents and the relative interviewed. It was also learned that Gary's father was working part-time and had not reported this income to Family Services. The guardian ad litem viewed the fact that Gary's father was working as a strength, even though the income earned was not reported.

The next step of working with Gary and his family involved linking them with needed social services. The guardian ad litem had to coordinate each of these services to ensure that the change effort was being followed through. It was decided that Gary should continue in foster care for two more months before his case would be reviewed. During this time, Gary would go into a special treatment program that would be aimed at increasing Gary's motor and intellectual development. Since the child was underweight and in the lower fifth percentile in height, regular visits to a medical doctor were prescribed. The guardian ad litem also instructed the foster parents to provide a stimulating environment for the child.

Gary's parents agreed to attend counseling for treatment of their alcohol problem. They also agreed to participate in parenting classes and were linked with other social services in the community. The guardian ad litem closely monitored the parents' activities to ensure that they followed through on the agreed plan. An effort was made to help Gary's father find a full-time job. The parents also agreed that when Gary visited each week for two hours they would not have relatives present. This strategy was used to help the guardian ad litem assess how the parents alone interacted with Gary.

After two months the guardian ad litem reassessed Gary's case. Gary's motor and intellectual development had improved through the efforts of the specialized treatment program and the foster parents. Gary was now able to walk alone and had a significant increase in his vocabulary. Gary's mother had followed through on her counseling for alcoholism; however, his father had missed a number of sessions. Gary's parents had also attended parenting classes on a regular basis. Gary's father found full-time employment. Since the income earned by Gary's father was extremely low, the family was eligible for a number of social services, including low-rent housing. During Gary's weekly two-hour home visits, only Gary's parents were present, and the guardian ad litem observed much improvement. Adequate housing and social services were obtained for the family. Gary also began receiving SSI because of his disability, fetal alcohol syndrome.

It was the opinion of the alcohol counselor that Gary's mother was making great progress; however, she was not deemed ready for Gary to return home. Some concern was also expressed about Gary's father not attending counseling on a regular basis. The professionals working with Gary, including the medical doctor, felt that Gary should continue to receive specialized treatment to improve his physical and emotional development. Thus it was decided that Gary should continue in foster care for two additional months. Gary's parents agreed to this plan. They would continue counseling, home visits would occur on a weekly basis for two hours, and Gary would continue receiving necessary treatment. This recommendation was made to the juvenile court and the judge agreed with the plan.

APPLICATION OF ADVOCACY TECHNIQUES TO GARY'S CASE

Fact Finding

Gary was placed in foster care because of child neglect. The neglect resulted in Gary being developmentally delayed physically and intellectually. He was also diagnosed with fetal alcohol syndrome; this syndrome contributed to his developmental delay. His parents were alcoholics. His father was working part-time. Gary's parents had limited parenting skills and were in need of comprehensive social services.

System Linking

Part of the advocacy process included the guardian ad litem linking Gary and his parents with needed social services. While in foster care, Gary received special treatment aimed at improving his motor and intellectual development. Gary also had regular visits with a medical doctor because of his failure to thrive and to treat problems related to his fetal alcohol syndrome. Gary's foster parents were also instructed to provide a stimulating environment, with the goal of improving his motor and intellectual development.

Needs Determination

The guardian ad litem was instrumental in helping Gary and his parents find needed social services. The advocate's efforts in this area resulted in improving the child's overall development. His parents also improved their parenting skills because of these services. Even though Gary and his parents were making significant improvements in a number of areas, the guardian ad litem advocated for Gary to remain in foster care and to continue to receive specialized services aimed at improving his motor and intellectual development.

Child Involvement

Gary did not possess the cognitive and intellectual development to participate in the treatment and advocacy process.

Developing Objectives

The objectives of Gary's case included continued placement in foster care until his parents were able to care for him properly. The guardian ad litem advocated for Gary and his parents to continue to receive needed social services during his placement in care. Particular emphasis in the case plan was for Gary to continue to have regular visits with a medical doctor in order to monitor his motor and intellectual development and to treat other medical problems related to his fetal alcohol syndrome.

Resolving Conflict

The need for conflict resolution by the guardian ad litem never occurred while working with Gary and his parents.

Implementing a Plan

The guardian ad litem advocated for Gary to remain in foster care until his parents were able to care for him and to meet his many needs. The permanency plan for Gary was to provide him with needed social and medical services, with the goal of returning him to his biological parents.

Protecting Children's Rights

The guardian ad litem helped to ensure that Gary received the protection of the juvenile court. Even though the goal was to return Gary to his biological parents, this was not going to occur until Gary's parents were able to provide a home environment that enhanced Gary's growth and development and met his meets.

SUMMARY AND CONCLUSION

Advocacy is a critical strategy for bringing about social change. It is a strategy grounded in a social justice/social work perspective. Advocacy is aimed at bringing about positive change in social systems that deny people their basic rights; it is also aimed at expanding the opportunities of the oppressed (Alinsky, 1946). Furthermore, advocacy is a powerful tool for changing the social environments of clients, including the systems that prevent the growth and development of individuals. Advocacy is a critical job for those who wish to effectively bring about social change.

Even though numerous disability laws are in place, including the IDEA and ADA, public and private entities often attempt to avoid compliance with these laws. Civil rights laws are at times not followed because they contradict bureaucratic rules of organizations, and organizations often perceive these as contributing to added costs.

When systems fail to comply with civil rights law, advocacy is an important strategy for ensuring compliance with civil rights law.

This chapter offers strategies for empowering individuals with disabilities through advocacy efforts. Even though advocacy is a highly technical skill, it is a skill that needs to be mastered by oppressed people. Advocacy is particularly effective when professionals teach persons with disabilities how to advocate for themselves. The power of advocacy when used as a litigation strategy was also emphasized in this chapter. A number of court cases were presented that illustrate how litigation can enhance children's rights.

Chapter 8

Children's Rights:
Implications for Policy and Practice

In Chapter 1 it was concluded that one of the greatest threats to the rights of children is poverty. Children living below the poverty level in the United States often do not have access to basic supports, including health care, housing, and proper nutrition. Poverty is often associated with underachievement in school, gang violence, and high unemployment. Most children in other developed countries are provided basic supports through highly developed family policies such as those found in Europe. The enactment of a comprehensive family policy in the United States would greatly enhance the lives of children and would also help ensure that many of their basic rights, such as access to health care, are met.

This chapter focuses on the importance of developing family policy in the United States. A model family policy is presented; this policy is designed to provide needed supports to children and their families. It is also suggested that an ecological perspective grounded in systems theory appears to be one of the more useful strategies for assessing and treating families under pressure. An interactional family therapy approach, sometimes referred to as strategic or communication family therapy, is presented in this chapter (Whall, 1986). This form of family therapy appears to be an effective strategy for treating families under pressure because it is grounded in the ecological perspective. Since families under pressure do not respond well to psychodynamic approaches, holistic approaches such as interactional family therapy appear to be a useful treatment alternative. Interactional family therapy offers much to troubled families because it views problems confronting families as part of the larger social ecology. It is also an approach that clearly endorses the need for comprehensive family policy as a part of treatment intervention. The chapter ends with a discussion of an emerging practice perspective, family health. Family health practice has the potential to be one of the most effective policy-practice strategies for ensuring that children's rights and needs are realized at both the policy and practice levels.

FAMILY POLICY

Rapid social change in the United States has created new pressures on the family system that are reflected in an increasing number of divorces, inadequate child care for children of working parents, an economy that prevents large numbers of families from meeting their basic needs, and health care and social service systems that are inadequate for millions of families (Pardeck, 1999). The public is also reluctant to help families through state and national programs.

In Chapter 7, a number of barriers were identified that appear to prevent the development of a national family policy in the United States. These are (1) an emphasis on the individual over the family system, (2) a preference for minimal government intervention into family life, and (3) pluralism. The following provides a more in-depth analysis of each of these barriers.

The first barrier to family policy, the emphasis on the individual over the family system, is well entrenched in the American ethos. Individuals have been encouraged to break away from their families of origin and shape their own destinies in accordance with personal merit. This tradition is consistent with the American economic and political systems (Pardeck, 1999).

Individualism has also shaped the perception of policymakers in defining social problems. Most social programs attempt to solve problems through changing individuals rather than the social structures that contribute to personal problems. This approach to problem solving has resulted in social policies and programs that deal with societal problems mainly at the individual level. Critics of this approach argue that individuals cannot change unless corresponding change occurs in the social systems that affect their social functioning.

The second barrier, the preference for minimal government intervention into family life, is ingrained in American culture. The view held by many citizens is that the home and family are bastions of privacy. It is also assumed that government intervention is counterproductive to family well-being.

The reluctance to intervene into family life is also grounded in the U.S. Constitution. The Constitution is completely silent on the subject of the family. Consequently, the implicit contract in American society is between the individual and the government. The Constitution's silence on the family has contributed to a void in the area of family policy.

The final barrier to family policy, pluralism, consists of the diverse beliefs, values, norms, and attitudes found in American society. Pluralism tends to thwart efforts to achieve consensus on policy and program development. For example, most Americans agree that a national health insurance program is needed; however, there is a lack of consensus on the components of the program and which level of government should administer the program (Karger and Stoesz, 2001).

Pluralism also contributes to the incremental development of policy and program development. Incrementalism involves compromise for consensus building and makes it nearly impossible to develop comprehensive and rational policies. Lindblom (1959) argues that the limits of human intelligence and current technology prevent comprehensive policy development. However, many Western societies have been able to develop efficient comprehensive social policies, including family policies, that include nationalized health care programs, as found in most European countries. These examples suggest that policy development and enactment can be comprehensive and effective (Pardeck, 1999).

Toward a National Family Policy

Advocates for a national family policy in the United States agree that the components of such a policy should include national health care, a comprehensive income assistance program, and social services (Pardeck, 1999). Given the incremental nature of policy development in the United States, a number of existing programs might be modified into comprehensive policies; these include health care programs, income supports, and social services.

Interest in a national health care program in the United States dates back to 1912, when the Progressive Party under Theodore Roosevelt included a national health care program in its platform. The original Social Security Act of 1935 included national health insurance, but it was removed to ensure passage of the Act (Jansson, 2005). Every

Congress since 1939 has introduced a national health care bill. President Truman in 1949 urged the enactment of a national health insurance system in his State of the Union message. The most recent effort to enact a national health care program occurred during the Clinton administration. The United States is one of the few industrialized nations that does not have a national health care program (Pardeck, 1999).

Support for national health care appears to be present and has been for some time. Medicare and Medicaid have the potential to serve as the foundation for a national health care program; however, the financing and operation of these two programs are entirely different. Medicare is basically a program for retired persons over the age of 65; it is financed through a premium paid by the insured and through the Social Security Act under Title 18. Medicaid is for the needy and low-income people; it is financed through federal and state governments as part of the Social Security Act under Title 19. Rather than creating an entirely new program, the Medicare and Medicaid programs could simply extend coverage to greater numbers of citizens. The Children's Health Insurance Program (CHIP) enacted in 1997 makes modification to the Medicaid program that extends coverage to middle-income families who have children with preexisting medical conditions. These medical conditions preclude families from buying health insurance from private vendors (Karger and Stoesz, 2001). The CHIP suggests that modifications in programs such as Medicare and Medicaid may be a useful strategy for extending health care protection to all citizens and families in the United States.

The need for some form of family income support is critical. Emerging economic issues such as low wages and underemployment of workers have created new pressures on families. Advocates of a family policy believe that a guaranteed income program would help relieve some of the economic pressures facing families. The United States is the only developed nation that does not have a coordinated economic support program for families (Karger and Stoesz, 2001).

Efforts have been aimed at developing a type of guaranteed family income; one serious effort was made by the Nixon administration. In the early 1970s, President Nixon sent a proposal to Congress called the Family Assistance Plan (FAP); this proposal called for a guaranteed income for all families. The FAP passed the House of Representatives but was defeated in the Senate; however, what emerged as a compromise in the Congress was a form of guaranteed income titled Supplemental Security Income (SSI). SSI provides a guaranteed income for people in certain categories, including the aged, persons with disabilities, and other dependent populations. The SSI program ensures a minimum income level for these groups. The program affects some families, mainly low-income; however, it is designed basically to meet individual needs. SSI might serve as the foundation for a guaranteed income program for families. Since the SSI program is already national in scope, the major policy modification in SSI would be to open program eligibility to families falling below a certain income level. The purpose of the program would be to ensure that no family's income is below a minimum level (Pardeck, 1999).

The final component of a national family policy, comprehensive social services, would have to be designed to meet the unique characteristics of American society. Since a national social services program for families would be difficult to regulate and coordinate, an innovative approach would have to be implemented. A voucher system has been suggested as one possible strategy for delivering social services to families (Karger and Stoesz, 2001).

A Model National Family Policy

Keeping these points in mind, a model family policy should include the following (Chung and Pardeck, 1997):

1. A decent standard of living for all children and families. This standard of living should be created through strategies aimed at creating jobs in the private and public sectors. Every head of a household should have access to work. If a household head is not able to work, the family should be provided a livable income.
2. Comprehensive health care for all families is imperative. This program would include children and their parents. The program must emphasize total health care by stressing the importance of diet, environment, and prevention. The program would be designed to keep families together during a health crisis. Presently, exorbitant health care costs create tremendous income pressures on many families.

3. Comprehensive social services must be made available to families. Many of the current problems facing families could be solved if services were available to them. Services should include child care, counseling services, and services for special problems, including permanent or temporary separation from the family. Comprehensive social services would be a departure from traditional approaches to assisting the family, which are mainly in the form of economic supports, such as public welfare.

4. The policy must provide for expanded research on family issues. This research would identify family needs. The research would emphasize three main areas:
   a. research on families in natural settings,
   b. systematic experimentation with and evaluation of children and family programs, and
   c. the development of social indicators reflecting the well-being of children and their families.

The research would help our understanding of the problems facing families and would offer solutions to these problems.

SOCIAL WORK PRACTICE AND CHILDREN

Social work practice with children is enhanced when it is grounded in an ecological perspective. The ecological perspective has tremendous utility for practice because it helps integrate policy with practice. The following presents an overview of the ecological perspective. Later in this section is a discussion of how policy and practice can be integrated through interactional family therapy.

Ecological Perspective

The ecological perspective explains human behavior in the context of social systems and the environment. The ecological perspective is a holistic orientation to assessment and treatment that includes the individual, family, organizational setting, community, and the larger social ecology. Assumptions guiding the ecological perspective include (Meinert, Pardeck, and Kreuger, 2000):

1. Transactions are understood as being contingent upon reciprocal exchange; transactions are the guide for understanding human behavior.
2. Life stress can be seen as positive or negative; life stressors create changes in the person-environment relationship.
3. Coping is viewed as part of the problem-solving process and helps to manage dysfunctional behavior.
4. Habitat is the social setting in which individuals function.
5. Niche is the result of one's accommodation to the environment.
6. Relatedness in one's environment supports attachments within the larger social ecology.

Systems Theory

A core theoretical grounding of the ecological perspective is systems theory. Systems theory helps practitioners understand how the client system functions in the larger social ecology. As a theoretical approach, it moves practitioners from a reductionistic view of human behavior to one stressing wholeness as the key to understanding individual behavior. Assumptions of systems theory include:

1. Wholeness suggests that change in one part of a system causes changes and modifications throughout a system.
2. Inputs regulate a system.
3. Equifinality suggests more than one way exists to get to a final system state.
4. Circular causality is not based in cause-and-effect relationships. Linear thinking as a guide to understanding human behavior has many limitations.

Practice Focus

The ecological perspective, with its emphasis on systems theory, provides the following guidelines for practice:

1. Transaction between the individual and family are critical for understanding human behavior.
2. The person in the environment is the context for practice.

3. An important aspect of practice is to focus on transitions through-out the life cycle.
4. The focus is on the strength of clients and families.
5. Assessment and intervention includes micro-, mezzo-, and macro-levels.

Limitations of the Ecological Approach

The limitations of the ecological perspective include:

1. The individual and family system must adapt to the environment; this adaptation may be oppressive to clients and families.
2. Change may be viewed as negative to the functioning of a system because homeostasis is a goal of intervention.
3. Systems have the potential to subordinate individuals, families, and autonomy.
4. The empirical evidence supporting the effectiveness of the ecological approach is limited. A number of disciplines, such as sociology, provide indirect evidence for the effectiveness of the ecological perspective as a grounding for assessment and intervention.

Given these limitations, the ecological systems perspective is a comprehensive perspective offering practice guidelines for assessment and intervention at multiple levels.

Family Therapy

Family therapy offers a viable treatment approach for those working with children and families. Most family therapy approaches are grounded to some degree in systems theory. The assumptions guiding systems theory were offered earlier in this chapter.

By grounding family therapy in systems theory, the focus of treatment moves from the individual to the family system. This notion was and continues to be revolutionary to the field of mental health. Many of the basic tenets guiding mainstream psychological theory have been challenged by the field of family therapy.

The grounding for systems theory found within the various approaches to family therapy can be traced to nineteenth-century sociologists and biologists (Timasheff, 1967). Modern-day systems theory has changed somewhat from its inception; however, the core assumptions underpinning systems theory remain the same. These include: (1) systems theory places great importance on interaction and interdependence of the parts of a system—change in one part of the system produces change in another part; (2) the effects of the social environment on individual social functioning is heavily emphasized; and (3) systems theory redefines the focus of pathology from the individual level to the systems level.

By using a systems approach to therapy, family therapists are able to better assess the impact of factors not always considered in individual treatment, including the influence of the social environment on individual social functioning. The individual-based therapies largely assume that the client is able to deal with pressures external to the self through treatment. As reviewed in Chapter 6, the empirical support for the efficacy of individual-based therapy is not impressive.

Empirical evidence for the effectiveness of family therapy as a treatment approach is also limited. Not that family therapy has been found to be ineffective, rather, limited effort has been made to test its effectiveness (Whall, 1986). This present limitation does not mean that practitioners should not use family therapy in treatment. Most therapeutic approaches are never tested empirically; however, efforts should be made to evaluate the effectiveness of family therapy to increase its legitimacy as a practice approach.

Interactional Family Therapy

Interactional family therapy incorporates a number of notions that appear critical to working effectively with children and their families. These include the ecological and systems perspectives. Interactional family therapists focus on communication patternings in the family system. They focus on how messages are sent and received by family members and the paths of communication within the family. Communication takes two forms, verbal and nonverbal. The famous concept within the field of family therapy, "double bind," was derived from research on family communication processes (Pardeck, 1981).

Interactional family therapists have completely divorced themselves from traditional psychological theories. Personality is seen as a result of interaction and transaction within the family and other systems. The intrapsychic is not considered important to the interactional family therapists because they view behavior as emerging from the transactional process with other systems, not from within the self (Whall, 1986).

Haley and Satir are representatives of interactional family therapy. Haley (1977), like Satir, argues that individual-based treatment approaches are largely ineffective because they do not consider the role of systems on human behavior. He suggests that therapists of the psychodynamic bent are no longer using a viable treatment model because the social ecology of individuals and families are not considered in intervention. Haley concludes that pathology is located in the family system, not the family member. Haley feels that psychopathology is a product of power struggles between individuals. This shift from conflict within the self to conflict outside the self challenges the essence of psychiatric theory.

Satir (1967) felt that we are all involved in multiple relationship systems and that our self-concepts and images are a result of interaction and transaction with social systems, particularly the family system. Satir (1967) also deemphasized the limitations of individual-based treatment modalities. She viewed problems as systems based, not individual based. She also placed great emphasis on family communication processes in her treatment approach. Satir felt that an important goal of treatment is to change these processes that are dysfunctional for the family system and its members.

According to Jones (1986), interactional family therapy uses a holistic approach to assessment and intervention that includes the following:

1. Assessment of the family structure including parents, children, personality and education levels of family members, and information on the extended family.
2. Social variables that need to be included in assessment are of the socioeconomic status of the family, religion, ethnicity, and the relationship of the family to the community.
3. A presenting problem is assessed from the perspective of each family member. What they feel will solve the problem is important to the assessment process. An analysis of family subsystems is included.
4. Communication processes are assessed. These include who speaks to whom, when, and in what tone. Family themes and

emotional climate help define how family members communicate with one another.

5. Role relationships are assessed; these include how supportive family members are of one another. Family coalitions, praising, and triangles are also analyzed.
6. Family developmental history is part of the assessment process. This includes information on the parents' families of origin. Developmental history of children and role relationships in the family over time are assessed.

Families who are at risk often need help in a number of the assessment areas previously listed. These include family communication, role relationships, and family developmental history. What is particularly important to the interactional family therapy assessment process is the inclusion of social variables. These variables are part of the ecological context that transacts with the family system.

Toward an Ecological Perspective

Many practitioners, particularly in the field of social work, use systems-based approaches to assess and treat families under pressure. The ecological perspective helps to broaden systems-based thinking because it includes the larger social ecology encompassing systems. The ecological perspective stresses the relationship between organisms and their social environment. It is a perspective that focuses heavily on the macrolevel by emphasizing the effects of the community, social organizations, and groups, including the family group, on individual behavior. It views traditional psychological theories as having limited utility for explaining human behavior. It is an approach that has synthesized knowledge from a number of disciplines. Interactional family therapy is based on the ecological perspective. The ecological perspective provides the practitioner with a more complete picture of family functioning. It also pushes the family practitioner to consider not only the effects of the family system on the individual but also the effects of the social environment on family functioning. One of several assumptions underpinning the ecological perspective that are built into interactional family therapy is the importance of the social environment on family functioning. The ecological perspective and interactional family therapy have a similar orientation toward social problems; that being social problems flow from the environment, not from the individual.

Haley, more so than other interactional family therapists, places great emphasis on the ecological perspective in treatment (Pardeck, 1981). Haley concludes that if therapists had total freedom they would work in their offices, their homes, in places of business, on the streets, or, for a school problem, in schools. Haley argues that therapists should think in organizational terms when providing treatment. The following quote, even though written several decades ago, summarizes the integration of interactional family therapy with the ecological perspective:

> What family therapists most have in common they also share with a number of behavioral scientists in the world today; there is an increasing awareness that psychiatric problems are social problems which involve the total ecological system. There is a concern with, and an attempt to change, what happens with the family, its interlocking systems, and the social institutions in which it is imbedded. The fragmentation of the individual, or the family, into parts is being abandoned. There is a growing consensus that a new ecological framework defines problems in new ways, and calls for new ways in therapy. (Haley, 1977, pp. 166-167)

Haley captures the essence of how one combines micro- and macro-levels of intervention. It offers a clear linkage between policy and practice with treatment intervention. Haley clearly argues that ideally, treatment should occur at multiple levels.

Family Therapy and Family Policy

The family system cannot be effectively treated unless the social environment is considered; the ecological perspective provides a framework for combining family intervention with policy (Pardeck, 1982). The ecological approach suggests that a comprehensive family policy is needed to help ensure children and families are provided with needed economic and social supports. A highly developed, comprehensive family policy can be viewed as an adjunct to the practitioner's treatment process. In fact, with such a policy, many families would never need treatment and those that are in treatment would have access to critical economic and social supports (Pardeck, 1999).

Minuchin and the Wiltwyck School for Boys (1967) demonstrate how family programs can assist family therapists in working with low-income families. Minuchin focuses on the unique pressures on low-income families and concludes that many problems they face would be relieved or eliminated if, during the treatment process, family programs such as day care and health services were made available to them.

Similar pressures also can be found in many families not confronted with poverty. One excellent example is the lack of quality day care available to middle-class families. Middle-class families, as well as all families, need quality day care in order to provide continuity of care to children. Numerous other programs would benefit families as well, such as parent education, comprehensive services for families of special needs children, and other related programs.

Comprehensive social services as an intricate part of family policy would help create an ecological environment conducive to family functioning. These kinds of social services and other supports would enhance the lives of children and families.

FAMILY HEALTH AND CHILDREN

Family health is an emerging practice orientation in the fields of social work, psychology, and other related disciplines. Social work has placed a great deal of emphasis on the family system since its inception; one could argue that the early roots of family health can be found in this profession. Given the fact that family health is a new innovation to a number of fields, the following serves as a guiding definition for this emerging practice approach:

> Family health is a state of holistic well-being of the family system. Family health is manifested by the development of, and continuous interaction among, the physical, mental, emotional, social, economic, cultural, and spiritual dimensions of the family which results in the holistic well-being of the family and its members. (Yuen and Pardeck, 1999, p. 1)

This section describes the philosophical basis of family health and offers the theoretical underpinnings of this innovative approach to intervention. Family health represents a distinct departure from the traditional medical model that has dominated the fields of medicine and mental health. The following discussion offers the basic premises guiding family health practice (Yuen and Pardeck, 1999).

Psychosocial Orientation

Family health is based on a psychosocial orientation to explaining human behavior. The traditional medical model assumes that pathology can be reduced to measurable biological variables; this view is inconsistent with the family health perspective. Even though the medical model has been very successful in treating numerous diseases, especially infectious diseases, the medical model has not been very useful for dealing with the complex social problems confronting clients and their families. Baird and Doherty (1990) suggest that the medical model represents nothing more than a cultural bias disguised as science.

The family health approach to practice views the problems of clients and their families within a larger social ecology. The practitioner grounded in the family health approach considers not only individual-based factors related to social functioning but also the family, community, and social context of the person in the environment. The focus of family health intervention includes the interaction and transaction of the family system within the larger social ecology. The locus of the family health approach is not the deficits or disease of the individual, but rather the promotion and maintenance of the total well-being of the individual in the family system (Yuen and Pardeck, 1999).

Focus of Practice

Family health practice focuses on the family as the most important context in which problems occur. A family health approach to practice emphasizes not only the biopsychosocial model but also the context in which problems occur. Four concepts are critical to this perspective (Pardeck and Yuen, 1997).

First, the family is the primary source of beliefs about health and behavior. The family also influences health-related behaviors. Minuchin (1974) helped identify the linkage between physical illness and family functioning. He found that family systems characterized as enmeshed, overprotective, and rigid often foster psychosomatic physical illness. Baird and Doherty (1990) report that many behaviors related to health are developed within the context of the family system, including smoking, diet, and exercise.

Second, stress on families can be manifested in social and physical symptoms; many stressors are related to life events. Life events include marriage, birth of a child, adolescence, leaving home, midlife crisis, death of a family member, and retirement (Carter and McGoldrick, 1988). Campbell (1986) also reports that illnesses increase when individuals are confronted with life stressors.

Third, social functioning can serve as an adaptive function for the family. Psychological problems can be understood as a barometer of the stress levels in a family system. For example, alcoholism can be viewed as a pathology that maintains the homeostasis in dysfunctional families. When the alcoholic improves, some family members may be threatened by the person moving out of the sick person role. This means the family must change, and change is a threat to dysfunctional families.

Fourth, families are one of the most important resources for family members under pressure. The family health practitioner realizes the tremendous support that families provide to family members who are experiencing problems. The family health practitioner uses the supportive functions of the family system by ensuring that family members are involved in all aspects of the assessment and treatment process (Pardeck and Yuen, 1997).

A family health approach to practice requires collaboration between practitioners and allied professionals. Practitioners must realize that they cannot meet all the needs of a family system under pressure. Many problems confronting family systems require the help of other professionals. It is critical for practitioners grounded in family health practice to develop positive relationships with allied professionals. This collaboration with others enhances the delivery of services to families in treatment (Yuen and Pardeck, 1999).

Practitioners using a family health approach view themselves as "a part of" rather than "apart from" the treatment process. Interventions such as the medical model view the practitioner as an objective outsider who diagnoses and treats problems. When treatment based in the medical model does not work effectively, the practitioner may blame the client and label him or her as "noncompliant." A family health approach to practice encourages practitioners to be sensitive to how their behavior influences the treatment process; this kind of reflective process enables the practitioner to be more responsive to the needs of clients and their families (Yuen and Pardeck, 1999).

What is powerful about the family health approach to practice is the large body of empirical research that provides support for it (Yuen and Pardeck, 1999). This literature illustrates the profound effect that the family system has on the physical and emotional health of family members. The holistic nature of family health ensures that practitioners assess and treat families' problems at both the policy and practice levels. Assessment and treatment are at multiple levels because family health considers a number of factors reflecting the health and well-being of family members and the family system; these include the physical, mental, emotional, social, economic, cultural, and spiritual dimensions of the family system. These factors must be treated at both the micro- and macrolevels. Effective family policy and programs are critical to the health of the family system.

Effective family policy influences the social, economic, cultural, and spiritual dimensions of family life. Healthy families enhance the lives of children; this notion obviously has tremendous implications for advocates in the field of children's rights.

Table 8.1 presents a comparison of family health practice with the medical model. Many traditional treatment modalities are grounded in the medical model. The medical model is representative of a number of individual-based treatment approaches that view the person as the cause and focus of social problems. As mentioned earlier in this chapter, individual-based treatments have minimal positive effect on family-based problems. Table 8.1 illustrates the critical differences between family health and the medical model.

A family health approach to practice has the potential to enhance the lives of children and families. It includes both micro- and macrolevels for understanding the health of the family system. As can be seen in Table 8.1, ill health is viewed as an imbalance of the family with the environment, the causes of ill health are multiple, and the health of families is a public concern. As stressed throughout this chapter, comprehensive family policy would greatly enhance the lives of children and their families.

TABLE 8.1. Assumptions of the Medical Model and Family Health Approaches

Concept	Medical Model Approach	Family Health Approach
Emphasis	Treating disease	Promotion of family health
Orientation	Disease approach	Ill health of families is an expression of imbalances in the ecological system
Causality	Locate causes in biochemical and organic functioning of body	Identify patterns among multi-levels of influence (holistic)
Intervention	Externally instigated	Enhancing internal capacity for healing
Professional's	Externally produced cure	The practitioner is a role facilitator of the healing process
Client's role	Passive	Active participant in the healing process
Society's role	Disease is a private industry	Family health and creating healthy environments is the public's responsibility

Source: Adapted from Weick (1986), The philosophical context of a health model of social work. *Social Casework* 67(9), pp. 551-559.

FAMILY HEALTH AND BIBLIOTHERAPY

Bibliotherapy can be a useful approach for helping children deal with psychological problems and various transitions through the family and individual life cycle. Bibliotherapy means helping clients, including children, deal with emotional and adjustment problems, as well as basic developmental needs, through the use of literature (Pardeck and Pardeck, 1989). Bibliotherapy can help children better verbalize their thoughts and feelings about confronting problems. Books can also help children find alternative solutions to problems through selected children's literature. Through reading literature, children can discover how others similar to themselves confronted problems and solved them. An in-depth review of the research literature by Pardeck and Pardeck (1989) concludes that bibliotherapy can help promote personal growth and development in children, promote social development, and help children deal with various psychological problems. These are all goals consistent with the family health perspective.

Bibliotherapy: Clinical Applications with Children in Foster Care and Adoption

The focus of this discussion is on the clinical applications of bibliotherapy. It will provide the clinical strategies for using fiction. The reader must keep in mind that bibliotherapy exists as a tool within the many spheres of therapy. It should be recognized that bibliotherapy is largely viewed as an adjunct to other therapeutic interventions. It would be unwise to look only to bibliotherapy as a sole cure in therapy (Shrodes, 1949, 1961). Just giving a child, for example, a book to read about a presenting problem does not cure the problem. The child must also be guided through the process of bibliotherapy by a trained practitioner. Keeping these points in mind, the following will overview strategies for using bibliotherapy through fiction, present how books are used in treatment, and offer techniques for matching books with children.

Effective Bibliotherapy

The following covers a number of critical issues designed to help ensure that successful bibliotherapy occurs. These include timing, book discussion, and the obligations of the practitioner.

Timing

Timing is a critical aspect of the bibliotherapeutic process. When a client is confronted with a presenting problem, he or she may not be ready to deal with it immediately. For example, a child who has been placed in foster care may not wish to deal with the emotional trauma of placement until he or she is emotionally ready. The practitioner may instead suggest to the foster parents that they have a book about a child in foster care, along with other reading materials, available in the home. In time, the child makes the decision to read or not read the book. A critical role of the practitioner in this process is to ensure that the book is appropriate for the special needs of the child. Techniques for identifying appropriate books to meet children's needs are discussed later in this chapter (Rudman, Gagne, and Bernstein, 1993).

The practitioner must realize that if a book is offered to the child at an inappropriate time, this action may intensify the problem or the child may become defensive. This tension within the client may prevent the book from influencing attitudes or behaviors. The child may respond to the book in such a way that he or she misses the point of the book and the positive strategies offered to resolve the problem.

If the practitioner allows children in particular to make their own book selections, guessing about the time will not be an issue. By allowing children to choose, practitioners need to be aware of the children's general background; this knowledge decreases the possibility of offending children on emotional, religious, moral, or other grounds.

Practitioners can facilitate self-selection by providing the means to attract children to relevant books for intervention. One strategy might be to decorate bulletin boards in the practitioner's office with book jackets from appropriate books for treatment. It might even be useful to have the book or books out on a table in the clinician's office. More discussion follows on timing in the next section of this chapter (Rudman, Gagne, and Bernstein, 1993).

Book Discussion

Skilled practitioners should be sensitive to the definite, overt, and clearly stated signs that children are amenable to having a book about a problem given to them. At the appropriate time, the practitioner provides the child with a book. After the child has read the book, in most circumstances it is advisable that the practitioner discuss the book with the child. Even though children gain some insight while reading alone, discussion is critical because it helps the child to explore in greater detail issues related to a presenting problem. However, just as the practitioner does not force a book on a child, the practitioner also should not intrude with unwanted discussion (Rudman, Gagne, and Bernstein, 1993).

Three dynamic interactions must take place for bibliotherapy to be successful; these include (Moody and Limper, 1971):

1. The author of a book must communicate clearly with the reader.
2. The client's ability to understand and respond to the material in the book is critical to successful bibliotherapy.
3. The practitioner must have the ability to perceive alterations in the client's attitudes and to bring those changes to a level of awareness in the client.

Certain things can be done to accomplish these objectives. One important action is for the practitioner to listen, instead of pushing the child to give reasons for choosing a book or offering analysis of the book. As in all sound therapeutic approaches, the practitioner must have sound listening skills.

When listening it is critical for the practitioner to use empathy in an appropriate way. An empathic relationship is generous. In an empathic relationship the practitioner's principle concern is encouraging the client to sustain and express his or her feelings and fantasies. Through empathy, the practitioner is able to perceive changes in attitudes and behaviors in the client.

When a practitioner listens with empathy, children in particular are offered the maximum opportunity to express their feelings. It allows children to trust and also provides cues when attitudes are changing. When the practitioner listens to the child, he or she will know how to react to the various verbal and nonverbal messages the child is sending. This helps the practitioner to gain insight into what areas should be covered with the child and what should be avoided. This process will also help to ensure that the appropriate books are used in treatment (Rudman, Gagne, and Bernstein, 1993).

Obligations of the Practitioner

Good timing and skillful listening are not the only important elements to the bibliotherapeutic process; it is also critical to realize that bibliotherapy demands that certain obligations must be met by the practitioner (Rudman, Gagne, and Bernstein, 1993).

The first obligation of the practitioner is to be familiar with the book before using it in treatment. Critical questions to explore when reviewing the book include the book's scope, its accuracy, its moral viewpoint, and whether it is worthwhile reading. Once these basic issues have been explored, the practitioner must examine the book's interest and reading levels, its format, length, and whether it is offered in other forms, such as large print.

The practitioner must also have an understanding of the child's reading abilities, general background, potential disabilities, and whether the child even enjoys reading or not. This information is critical to the book-selection process.

The practitioner must of course have good clinical skills. These include warmth, empathy, and being able to assess the effectiveness of the use of books in treatment. Positive therapeutic outcome when using bibliotherapy typically means the relationship between the practitioner and the client is built on trust and warmth. The practitioner must also keep in mind that bibliotherapy is an adjunct to treatment, not the core treatment.

The following questions might be helpful to explore when choosing books for treatment; these questions are framed for choosing books for children in foster care or adoptive placement:

1. Is the book an appropriate fit for the foster or adoptive home?
2. Will the book on foster care or adoption cause more problems than it will solve?
3. Will the book offend the foster or adoptive child's family on religious or moral grounds? If so, what should be done to correct this situation?
4. Should the book on foster care or adoption be read in a group setting?
5. Will children who have not experienced foster care or adoption, but who will have such an experience in the future, be frightened by the book?
6. On the contrary, should children who have encountered placement be protected from a discussion about the placement process in a book?
7. Should a book on placement in foster care or adoption be graphic about these experiences or should the book present the process of placement through metaphors?

The basic obligations of the practitioner using bibliotherapy can be realized by exploring these questions and issues. Furthermore, the practitioner will use bibliotherapy with greater confidence when working with children in foster care or adoption when these questions are thoroughly explored.

Using Bibliotherapy with Fiction

Figure 8.1 illustrates the procedures for using bibliotherapy with fictional books; however, some nonfiction works can also be utilized with this approach (Pardeck and Pardeck, 1983, 1987, 1989). The bibliotherapeutic process presented in Figure 8.1 offers a series of distinct activities that are critical to using books in therapy. These include the child's readiness and book selection, as well as the child actually reading the book. The bibliotherapeutic process also calls for meaningful follow-up activities. These activities are aimed at moving the child through the stages of the bibliotherapeutic process.

Readiness

Before proceeding with the bibliotherapeutic process, the therapist must consider an important factor—the child's readiness for bibliotherapy. Inappropriate timing may impede the process. Typically, the child is ready for the initiation of bibliotherapy when the following conditions have been met:

1. Rapport, trust, and confidence have been established between the practitioner and the child.
2. The child and practitioner have agreed on the presenting problem(s).
3. Preliminary exploration of the problem has occurred (Zaccaria and Moses, 1968).

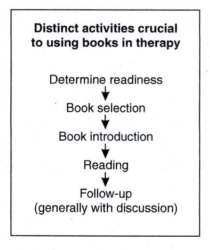

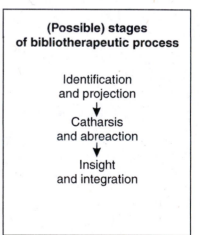

FIGURE 8.1. Aspects of Treatment Approach to Bibliotherapy (The activities are set steps that must occur in order. The stages of the process are more approximate—each child will progress through these stages at different rates, both during and after reading the book.)

Selection of Books

The practitioner must consider several factors when identifying books for treatment. The most important factor is the presenting problem(s) of the child. The child may be confronted with a minor or major adjustment problem (Coleman and Ganong, 1990). Although books are available on virtually any topic, it is essential when using books in treatment that the work contain believable characters and situations that offer realistic hope for the child. The practitioner must also know the child's interests and reading level. One additional element in selection is the book's form of publication. Alternative forms such as braille, talking books (cassettes or CDs), and large print are available for special needs children. The practitioner may wish to use a paperback edition when working with older children (Pardeck and Pardeck, 1989).

Introducing the Book

When the child is ready for the bibliotherapeutic process to begin and book selection has been completed, the therapist's next concern is how to introduce the book into treatment. Most practitioners feel that it is best to suggest books rather than to prescribe them; however, one may have to prescribe books for very young children (Griffin, 1984). Regardless of what strategy the practitioner uses for introducing books into treatment, he or she must be familiar with the content of the books selected (Pardeck and Pardeck, 1998).

Follow-Up Strategies

Zaccaria and Moses (1968) conclude that most studies dealing with the use of books in treatment suggest that the reading of a book must be accompanied by discussion. During and after reading the book, the child may experience the three stages of the bibliotherapeutic process: Identification and Projection, Catharsis and Abreaction, and Insight and Integration (Orton, 1997). Obviously, very young children are not capable of experiencing abreaction and catharsis leading to insight into a presenting problem in the traditional therapeutic sense. For older children, the advanced stages of the bibliotherapeutic process are important for successful treatment when using fiction and certain kinds of nonfiction books (Pardeck and Pardeck, 1998).

Books on Foster Care

Even though foster care is intended to be a temporary placement for children, many times it is not. Children who experience foster care often have a very predictable emotional and behavioral reaction to it. When placed, they feel separation and loss from their biological parents. They often protest against placement and do not understand why they had to be placed in foster care. Anger at and distrust of adults, particularly foster parents, is very common in foster children. Through support and understanding, most children can work through the emotional turmoil of placement in foster care. Most children can adjust to the reality of foster care; however, it is very difficult for them to grow and thrive in this kind of substitute care.

The annotated books listed here are examples of books that focus on the various kinds of problems children are confronted with in foster care. Each annotation describes the book. The following books are for junior high children and older.

1. Adler, C. *The Cat That Was Left Behind.* New York: Clarion, 1981.

    Chad Lester, a thirteen-year-old foster child, has been sent to another foster home. A parallel is drawn between thirteen-year-old Chad and a stray cat. As Chad tames the cat and cares for it, he gradually comes to terms with the facts he has long denied— that his unmarried mother who now has married does not want him back with her.

2. Bloomquist, G. and Bloomquist, P. *Coping As a Foster Child.* Placerville, CA: Rosen, 1992.

    Case studies of teenagers in foster care are presented, highlighting successes as well as failures in placement. Reasons behind placement are explored and a variety of placements are explained: therapeutic foster homes, adoption and rejections, and independent living programs. Facts are covered, yet the real-life emotions of teens in foster care are elaborated on.

3. Davies, N. M. *Foster Care*. New York: Watts, 1994.

The history of foster care, responsibilities of foster parents, and the preparation of caseworkers are discussed, as well as day-to-day life in a typical foster home. Different trends in social welfare policy and an explanation of the 1980 Adoption Assistance and Child Welfare Act are covered. Pros and cons of the foster care system are both presented.

4. Desetta, A. (Ed.). *The Heart Knows Something Different: Teenage Voices from the Foster Care System*. New York: Persea Books, 1996.

Fifty-seven essays explore a variety of feelings associated with teens who have been in foster care. Reasons why children are placed in care, self-awareness, and a sense of purpose in looking toward the future comprise the four sections of this book. Regret and remorse over the past is sometimes expressed; teenagers turning their lives around is a central theme.

5. Falke, J. *Everything You Need to Know About Living in a Foster Home*. Placerville, CA: Rosen, 1995.

Reasons that children must be placed in foster care are presented, as well as short anecdotes about abuse and neglect. Foster home standards are explained and the criteria for becoming foster parents are covered. Open communication, discussion of feelings, and developing trust with foster children are stressed.

6. Gay, K. *Adoption and Foster Care*. Springfield, NJ: Enslow, 1990.

A factual overview of both topics, stating that 6 million adoptees and several hundred thousand foster children are in the United States. The difference between foster care and adoption is provided, including a brief history, as well as the issues of open adoption and racially mixed foster and adoptive families. Caregiver anecdotes are provided.

Books on Adoption

Often when children are initially placed in adoption, they fantasize about returning to their biological parents. Once children realize that they are not returning to their birth parents, some will enter a period of mourning. Anger and emotional pain are often part of this process. Even though children in adoption may realize that they will not be returning to their parents, the fantasy is never completely given up.

The first week of placement in adoption often goes smoothly, but this "honeymoon" period is artificial. When adoptive children after initial placement begin longing for the past, feelings of emotional pain begin to emerge. Children may also fear that they will be rejected by their adoptive parents. This is an indication that children in adoption are beginning to bond with their new parents. Behavioral problems are likely at this stage of the adoption process. However, in due course many children gradually adjust to their new homes.

This annotated list provides examples of books on adoption. They focus on the typical reactions that children experience when placed in adoption. The books are for junior high children and older.

1. Arms, S. *Adoption: A Handful of Hope*. Berkeley, CA: Celestial Arts, 1989.

    This work contains a series of case studies that offer the personal and moving accounts of children who have been adopted, adoptive parents, and women who have given their babies up for adoption. The author attempts to show how the process of adoption can be improved for all parties involved.

2. Cohen, S. *Coping with Being Adopted*. New York: Rosen, 1988.

    The common problems associated with being adopted are discussed, and ways for coping with adoption are offered. The book includes sections on transracial and handicapped adoptees, as well as other issues related to the complexity of the adoption process.

3. Gay, K. *Adoption and Foster Care*. Springfield, NJ: Enslow, 1990.

    A factual overview of both topics, stating that 6 million adoptees and several hundred thousand foster children are in the United States. The difference between foster care and adoption is provided, including a brief history, as well as the issues of open adoption and racially mixed foster and adoptive families. Caregiver anecdotes are provided.

4. Gravelle, K. and Fischer, S. *Where Are My Birth Parents? A Guide for Teenage Adoptees*. New York: Walker Publishing Company, 1993.

    This is a self-help book designed to assist teenage children in their search for biological parents. The book stresses that the individual identity of adoptees can be enhanced through searching for their biological parents. The work offers the stories of three adopted children: Chloe, Emily, and Selena.

5. Holland, I. *The House in the Woods*. New York: Little, 1991.

The only adopted child in her family, fourteen-year-old Bridget wonders about her birth parents. She is overweight and must deal with her mother's death, as well as annoying younger siblings and an aloof nanny. A summer vacation reveals information about Bridget's birth and she eventually meets her alcoholic birth father.

6. Maguire, J. *Starting Over.* New York: Ballantine, 1992.

A wealthy teenage girl discovers she was adopted at birth and decides to seek out her biological mother. Her friends, who all have family problems of their own, all help with her search. The biological mother has little interest in being reunited with her daughter, who is one more reminder of her middle age. National hotline numbers are included.

FAMILY HEALTH AND CLINICAL ASSESSMENT

Family health social work practice is an intervention strategy that includes clinical aspects of family life not typically considered in other, more traditional approaches to family intervention. It is a holistic approach that focuses on the physical, mental, emotional, social, economic, cultural, and spiritual dimensions of the family system. Given this perspective, the assessment of the family system should include both micro- and macrolevel areas of family functioning. Microlevel areas include the physical, mental, and emotional aspects of family life; the macrolevel areas focus on the social, economic, and cultural aspects of family functioning. The following offers a number of clinical instruments that practitioners will find useful for assessing family health at both the micro- and macrolevels.

Assessment and Social Work Practice

Accurate assessment is important for effective social work intervention (Wodarski, 1981). This is particularly important to help ensure that children and their families receive accurate assessment to help ensure positive treatment outcome. A number of assessment instruments are currently available that involve little time, energy, or cost to administer. These instruments are designed to measure various factors that are critical to conducting an analysis of a client's presenting problem. They are designed to conduct assessment at the individual, family, and environmental levels. Many of these tools are also available in computer format, which increases their ease of use for practice. The following reviews a variety of assessment instruments currently available that will help facilitate assessment and treatment from a family health perspective (Pardeck, 1996).

The instruments presented include behavior rating scales, self-report inventories, structured interviews, and observational coding systems. Behavior rating scales are completed by an informed source in reference to behavioral characteristics of a client system, including a family system, whereas self-report inventories are completed by the client. Behavior rating scales and self-report inventories are easier to administer than the structured interview or direct observation. Behavior rating scales and self-report inventories provide empirical information about the success of an intervention (Pardeck, 1996).

Standardized questions and responses are a part of the structured interview, which provides extensive information on a client's social functioning. Observational coding systems involve observing and recording the frequency of certain behaviors and events in a naturalistic or structured situation. This approach involves a great deal of time and effort on the part of the practitioner (Pardeck, 1996).

Using and Selecting Instruments

For an instrument to effectively assess a presenting problem of a client, it must have acceptable levels of reliability and validity. The instruments offered here have acceptable reliability and validity. This means they consistently and accurately measure what they claim to measure (Pardeck, 1996).

The practitioner should become familiar with the assessment instruments prior to their use. Basic information on each instrument is offered, including what the instrument measures and the kind of client population the instrument is used to make assessments about (Pardeck, 1996).

When the practitioner uses assessment instruments, the client must give his or her informed consent. The client should be told what the instrument assesses and who will see the information generated from the assessment. If the practitioner keeps these important points in mind, the instruments should increase practice effectiveness (Pardeck, 1996).

Assessment at the Individual Level

The following instruments are available for conducting family health assessment regarding children and parental social functioning. They are largely designed to conduct assessment at the individual level.

Adolescent Alcohol Involvement Scale (Mayer and Filstead, 1979)

This fourteen-item self-report inventory categorizes adolescent alcohol use/abuse along a continuum from abstinence to misuse. It has demonstrated high test-retest reliability in screening adolescent populations for alcohol misuse.

Adult-Adolescent Parenting Inventory (Bavolek, 1984)

This is a thirty-two-item self-report inventory aimed at measuring parenting strengths and weaknesses in four areas: inappropriate developmental expectations, lack of empathy toward children's needs, belief in use of corporal punishment, and reversal of parent-child roles. The client responds to each item on a five-point scale (from "strongly agree" to "strongly disagree").

Beck Depression Inventory (Beck, 1967)

This consists of a twenty-one-item self-report inventory widely used in clinical practice for measuring depression. Clients indicate on a scale from zero to three the severity of their current symptoms.

Behavior Problem Checklist (Quay, 1977)

This fifty-five-item behavior-rating scale assesses the types and degree of behavioral problems in children and adolescents. The practitioner completes the three-point scale. The scale consists of four subscales, including identifying conduct problems, personality problems, inadequacy-immaturity, and socialized delinquency.

Child Behavior Checklist (Achenbach and Edelbrock, 1979)

This is a 118-item behavioral-rating scale widely used to measure problem behaviors of children. The practitioner rates a variety of behaviors on a three-point scale. These include the checklist measures for internalizing syndromes (i.e., depression, immaturity) and externalizing syndromes (i.e., aggression, hyperactivity).

Children's Beliefs About Parental Divorce Scale (CBAPDS)
(Kurdek and Berg, 1987)

This thirty-six-item assessment scale is designed to measure children's beliefs about their parents' divorce. The instrument uses a yes/no response format. It is designed for children ages eight to fourteen.

Children's Depression Inventory (Kovacs, 1981)

This twenty-seven-item self-report inventory is a modified version of the Beck Depression Inventory. It measures overt symptoms of childhood depression including sadness, suicidal ideation, and sleep and appetite disturbances. The inventory is designed for children ages eight to fourteen. The child responds to a three-point scale for each item.

Children's Cognitive Assessment Questionnaire (CCAQ)
(Zatz and Chassing, 1983)

This forty-item assessment instrument measures self-defeating and self-enhancing cognition associated with test anxiety and is useful for practitioners working in school or residential settings. It consists of a true/false format for each item and is designed for children ages nine to twelve.

Children's Perceived Self-Control (CPSC) Scale (Humphrey, 1982)

This eleven-item scale measures self-control from a cognitive-behavioral perspective. It is designed for children eight to twelve years of age. The scale addresses interpersonal self-control, personal self-control, and self-evaluation and uses a "usually yes" or "usually no" format for each item.

Depression Self-Rating Scale (DSRS) (Birleson, 1981)

This scale assesses the extent and severity of depression in children. The instrument consists of eighteen items and assesses depression in children between the ages of seven and thirteen. The instrument includes items on a three-point scale that assesses mood, physiological and somatic complaints, and cognitive aspects of depression.

Developmental Profile II (Alpern, Boll, and Shearer, 1980)

This 186-item behavioral-rating scale assesses the functioning of children from birth to age nine in five areas including physical, self-help, social, academic, and communication. The items are rated either "pass" or "fail." The scale can be completed in twenty to forty minutes by a practitioner employing knowledge of the child's skills, observations, and/or parent interviews.

Generalized Contentment Scale (Hudson, 1992)

This twenty-five-item self-report inventory, rated in a one-to-seven continuum, measures the degree, severity, and magnitude of non-psychotic depression and focuses largely on affective aspects of depression.

Implicit Parental Learning Theory Interview
(Honig, Caldwell, and Tannenbaum, 1973)

This forty-five-item, forty-five-minute structured interview is designed to inventory the techniques a parent uses to deal with developmentally appropriate behaviors of preschool children. Five forms are available for use with parents of children ages one to four and five to six.

Index of Self-Esteem (Hudson, 1992)

This twenty-five-item self-report inventory, rated on a one-to-seven continuum, measures the degree, severity, and magnitude of a client's problem in the area of self-esteem.

Index of Peer Relationships (Hudson, 1992)

This twenty-five-item self-report inventory, rated on a one-to-seven continuum, measures the degree, severity, and magnitude of a client's problems in relationships with peers. It can be used as a global measure of peer relationship problems in a number of settings.

Index of Sexual Satisfaction (Hudson, 1992)

This twenty-five-item self-report inventory, rated on a one-to-seven continuum, measures the degree, severity, and magnitude of sexual discord or dissatisfaction in a dyadic relationship.

Maternal Characteristics Scale (Polansky, Gaudin, and Kilpatrick, 1992)

This thirty-five-item observational rating scale consists of descriptive statements with which the practitioner assesses relatedness, impulse control, confidence, and verbal accessibility. The practitioner responds to true or false (or mostly true/mostly false) items.

Michigan Screening Profile of Parenting (Paulson, Afifi, Chaleff, Thomason, and Liu, 1975)

This thirty-item self-report inventory assesses attitudes regarding child rearing and parental self-awareness and self-control. Clients respond to each item on a seven-point scale ranging from "strongly agree" to "strongly disagree."

Nowicki-Strickland Locus of Control Scale (N-SLCS) (Nowicki and Strickland, 1973)

This forty-item scale is designed to assess a child's beliefs about chance or fate. Targeted for children eleven to eighteen years of age, the scale features items requiring a yes or no response.

Partner Abuse Scale: Non-Physical (PASNP) (Hudson, 1992)

This twenty-five-item self-report inventory, rated on a one-to-seven continuum, measures the degree, severity, and magnitude of nonphysical abuse from a spouse or partner.

Physical Abuse Partner Scale (PAPS) (Hudson, 1992)

This twenty-five-item self-report inventory, rated on a one-to-seven continuum, measures the degree, severity, and magnitude of physical abuse from a spouse or partner.

Problem-Oriented Screening Instrument for Teenagers (POSIT) (Rahdert, 1991)

This 139-item self-report screening instrument assesses substance-abuse problems, physical health status, mental health status, family relationships, peer relationships, educational status, vocational status, social skills, leisure and recreation, and aggressive behavior/delinquency. It is designed for children ages thirteen to nineteen years.

Rosenberg Self-Esteem Scale (Rosenberg, 1979)

This ten-item self-report inventory measures the self-esteem of children thirteen to eighteen years of age. The child rates each item on a four-point scale.

Self-Perception Profile for Children (Harter, 1982)

This twenty-eight-item self-rating inventory assesses cognitive, social, and physical competence in children. The scale is designed for children in the third through ninth grades. For each item, the child is asked to first identify which of two passages best describes the child, then the child rates whether the description is "sort of true" or "really true."

Assessment at the Family Level

The instruments that follow focus on family health assessment at the familial level and also address family functioning in marital relationships.

Attitude Toward the Provision of Long-Term Care (Klein, 1992)

This twenty-six-item self-report inventory, rated on a one-to-five continuum, assesses attitudes toward the provision of informal long-term care for family members.

Child's Attitudes Toward Mother (CAM) (Hudson, 1992)

This twenty-five-item self-report inventory, rated on a one-to-seven continuum, measures the degree, severity, and magnitude of problems a child has with his or her mother.

Child's Attitudes Toward Father (CAF) (Hudson, 1992)

This twenty-five-item self-report inventory, rated on a one-to-seven continuum, measures the degree, severity, and magnitude of problems a child has with his or her father.

Co-Dependency Inventory (CODI) (Stonebrink, 1988)

This twenty-nine-item instrument is designed to assess codependency in family and friends of substance abusers. Codependency is defined as enabling the abuser to continue to use chemicals and/or trying to control the abuser's use of alcohol and/or drugs. The client responds to items on a four-point continuum.

Conflict Tactics Scale (Straus, 1979)

This nineteen-item self-report inventory is used to assess conflict among family members. A parent or child responds to a six-point scale (from "never" to "more than twenty times") to indicate the number of times in the past year specific techniques were used during family conflict.

Dyadic Adjustment Scale (Spanier and Filsinger, 1983)

This thirty-two-item self-report inventory consists of three different types of rating responses measuring satisfaction in intimate relationships.

Dyadic Parent-Child Interaction Coding System
(Robinson and Eyberg, 1981)

This observational assessment tool assesses the interaction of parents and young, conduct-problem children. Parent and child are observed during fifteen-minute segments as they interact in three structured clinical situations.

Family Adaptability and Cohesion Evaluation Scales
(FACES III) (Olson, 1986)

FACES III is a forty-item self-report assessing the cohesion and adaptability of family functioning. Cohesion is defined as the degree of emotional bonding between family members; adaptability is defined as the ability of the family system to change its power structure, roles, and rules in response to environmental stress.

Family Assessment Device (FAD)
(Hendershot and LeClere, 1993)

FAD assesses family dynamics, which include affective involvement, behavioral control, roles, problem solving, communication, and affective responsiveness.

Family Assessment Form (McCroskey, Nishimoto,
and Subramanian, 1991)

This observational assessment tool includes five subscales with 102 items. It assesses the family's physical, social, and economic environment; psychosocial history of caregivers; personal characteristics of caregivers; child-rearing skills; caregiver-to-child interactions; developmental status of children; and overall psychosocial functioning of the family. Family functioning is rated on a five-point scale linked to child maltreatment.

Family Assessment Measure (FAM III)
(Hendershot and LeClere, 1993)

FAM III assesses the following family dynamics: affective involvement, control, role performance, task accomplishment, communication, affective expression, and values and norms.

Family Environment Scale (FES)
(Hendershot and LeClere, 1993)

The FES assesses three dimensions of family functioning: relationships, personal growth, and systems maintenance. The relationship dimension assesses family cohesion, expression, and conflict. The personal growth dimension assesses family independence, moral-religious emphasis, and a family's achievement, intellectual-cultural, and active-recreational orientation. The systems-maintenance dimension assesses the organization and control found within a family system.

Family Functioning Scale (FFS) (Hendershot and LeClere, 1993)

The FFS assesses the overall functioning of a family. Five dimensions are assessed; these include affect, family communication, family conflict, family worries, and family rituals/supports.

Index of Brother Relations (IBR) (Hudson, 1992)

This twenty-five-item self-report inventory, rated on a one-to-seven continuum, measures the degree, severity, and magnitude of problems a person has with his or her brother.

Index of Family Relations (Hudson, 1992)

This instrument assesses the extent, severity, and magnitude of problems that family members experience in a family system. It offers a global assessment of family relations. It employs a twenty-five-item self-report inventory rated on a one-to-seven continuum measuring the extent, severity, or magnitude of problems that family members have in their relationship with one another.

Index of Marital Satisfaction (Hudson, 1992)

This twenty-five-item self-report inventory, rated on a one-to-seven continuum, measures the degree, severity, and magnitude of problems with a spouse or partner.

Index of Parental Attitudes (Hudson, 1992)

This twenty-five-item self-report inventory, rated on a one-to-seven continuum, measures the extent, severity, and magnitude of parent-child relationship problems as perceived and reported by the parent in reference to a child.

Index of Sister Relations (ISR) (Hudson, 1992)

This twenty-five-item self-report inventory, rated on a one-to-seven continuum, measures the degree, severity, and magnitude of problems a person has with his or her sister.

Index of Spouse Abuse (Hudson and McIntosh, 1981)

This thirty-item self-report scale, rated on a one-to-five continuum, measures the severity and magnitude of physical or nonphysical abuse inflicted on a woman by her spouse or partner. Clinical cutting scores are recommended for both physical or nonphysical abuse subscale scores.

Inventory of Family Feelings (Lowman, 1980)

This thirty-eight-item self-report inventory assesses the overall degree of attachment between family members. Family members respond to a three-point scale on each item.

Marital Satisfaction Inventory (Snyder, 1983)

This 280-item self-report inventory assesses an individual's attitudes and beliefs regarding eleven specific areas of marital functioning. The inventory requires approximately thirty minutes for individual spouses to respond to true-false items and includes subscales on dissatisfaction with children and conflict over child rearing.

Parent-Adolescent Communications Inventory (Bienvenu, 1969)

This forty-item self-report inventory assesses communication patterns and characteristics between parents and adolescents. Adolescents aged thirteen to nineteen years respond to each item using a three-point scale.

Parent-Child Behavioral Coding System (Forehand and McMahon, 1981)

This observational tool assesses patterns of parent-child interaction. A practitioner codes parent and child behaviors in a ten-minute, structured exercise in a clinic setting or in a forty-minute unstructured home visit.

Parent Locus of Control Scale (PLOC) (Campis, Lyman, and Prentice-Dunn, 1986)

This forty-seven-item, five-point scale is designed to assess parental locus of control relating to the parent's (internal) or child's (external) power in a given family situation. Items assess parental efficacy, parental responsibility, child's control of parents' life, parental belief in fate and chance, and parental control of child's behavior.

Parental Authority Questionnaire (PAQ) (Buri, 1991)

This thirty-item assessment tool includes a five-point scale designed to measure parental authority and disciplinary practice.

Self-Report Family Inventory (SFI) (Olson and Tiesel, 1993)

The SFI is theoretically grounded in the Beavers Systems Model of Family Functioning (BSM) Two dimensions are measured: (1) overall competence and behavior of the family system and (2) emotional style used by the family system. The overall competence dimension includes family happiness, optimism, problem solving, and parental coalitions. The behavioral and emotional style dimension assesses family conflict, communication, cohesion, leadership, and emotional expression.

Standardized Observation System 3 (Wahler, House, and Stambaugh, 1976)

This observational tool assesses interactions between a child and other members of a family system. The practitioner codes the interactional sequence in a one-hour, unstructured home visit.

Environmental Level

The assessment instruments listed here focus on macrolevel analysis. Specifically, they assist the practitioner in assessing the family system as it interacts with the environment. This kind of assessment provides important information for conducting macrolevel family health intervention.

Child Abuse Potential Survey (Milner, Gold, Ayoub, and Jacewitz, 1984)

This 160-item self-report inventory, completed by a parent, is designed to be used as a screening device to differentiate physical abusers from nonabusers. Factors assessed include distress, rigidity, child with problems, problems from family and others, unhappiness, loneliness, and negative concepts of child and self. Respondents are asked either to agree or disagree with each item.

Child Well-Being Scales (Magura and Moses, 1986)

These forty-three behavior-rating scales are a multidimensional measure of child maltreatment situations specifically designed for use as an outcome measure in child protective services programs rather than for individual cases. The scales focus on actual or potential unmet needs of children. Current testing of the subscales indicates that three factors (household adequacy, ten scales; parental disposition, fourteen scales; and child performance, four scales) accounted for 43 percent variance and that the Child Well-Being Scale can discriminate between neglectful and nonneglectful families. It requires approximately twenty-five minutes for the practitioner to complete and is based on direct contact with the family, including in-home visits. Each dimension is rated on a three- or six-point continuum of adequacy/inadequacy.

Childhood Level of Living Scale (Polansky, Chalmers, Buttenwieser, and Williams, 1981)

This ninety-nine-item behavior-rating scale assesses neglect of children up to seven years of age. The nine subscales include: general positive child care, state of repair of home, negligence, quality of household maintenance, quality of health care and grooming, encouragement of competence, inconsistency of discipline and coldness, encouragement of superego development, and material giving. It requires approximately fifteen minutes for the practitioner who knows the family well to answer all items "yes" or "no."

Environmental Assessment Index (EAI) (Poresky, 1987)

This forty-four-item index (or twenty-two-item short form) is designed to assess the educational/developmental quality of children's home environments. A practitioner scores each yes-or-no item based on either direct observation or information from the child's parent.

Family Inventory of Life Events and Changes
(McCubbin and Patterson, 1983)

This seventy-one-item self-report inventory records normative and nonnormative stressors a family unit may experience within a year. Family members (together or separately) respond "yes" or "no" to each item. Norms are provided for families at various stages of the family life cycle.

Family Risk Scales (Magura, Moses, and Jones, 1987)

This scale consists of twenty-six behavioral-rating items designed to identify a full range of situations predictive of near-term child placement so that preventive services can be offered and change monitored. The scales are similar to the Child Well-Being Scales. Dimensions are focused on the areas that are potentially malleable.

Home Observation for Measurement of the Environment
Inventory (Caldwell and Bradley, 1978)

This 100-item observation/interview procedure inventory assesses the quality of stimulation of a child's early environment. Two versions of the inventory were designed: one for children aged birth to three years and one for three- to six-year-olds. Approximately one-third of the items are answered through a parent interview; the practitioner of the child and the primary caretaker in the home answers the remaining items on observations. It requires approximately one hour to answer all of the items with a "yes" or "no" response.

Inventory of Socially Supportive Behaviors (Barrera, Sandler, and Ramsay, 1981)

This forty-item self-report inventory assesses the frequency with which individuals have received aid and assistance from the people around them. Respondents answer each item through a five-point scale (from "not at all" to "every day").

Multi-Problem Screening Inventory (MPSI) (Hudson, 1990)

This is a 334-item self-report scale measuring twenty-seven dimensions of family functioning. Subscales measure the following: depression, self-esteem, partner problems, sexual discord, child problems, mother problems, personal stress, friend problems, neighbor problems, school problems, aggression, work associates, family problems, suicide, nonphysical abuse, physical abuse, fearfulness, ideas of reference, phobias, guilt, work problems, confused thinking, disturbing thoughts, memory loss, alcohol abuse, and drug abuse. Questions are answered through a seven-point Likert scale (from "none of the time" to "all of the time"). The scale can be computer-scored.

Parenting Stress Index (Abidin, 1986)

This 101-item self-report index assesses a mother's perception of stress associated with child and parent characteristics. An additional nineteen optional items can be administered assessing stressful life events. Mothers complete the index in approximately thirty minutes.

Provision of Social Relations (PSR) (Turner, Frankel, and Levin, 1983)

This fifteen-item instrument is designed to assess components of social support. The items are responded to through a five-point continuum. Social support includes attachment, social integration, reassurance of worth, reliable alliance, and guidance.

Social Support Behaviors Scale (Vaux, Riedel,
and Stewart, 1987)

This forty-five-item self-report inventory assesses five modes of support: emotional, socializing, practical assistance, financial assistance, and advice/guidance. Respondents record on a five-point scale (from "no one would do this" to "most family members/friends would certainly do this") the likelihood of family and friends helping in various ways.

SUMMARY AND CONCLUSION

This chapter focuses on strategies for combining policy and practice. It is concluded that a comprehensive family policy would help prevent many of the problems that plague children and families within the United States. Family policy is particularly needed for combating one of the greatest threats to the rights of children: poverty.

An ecological perspective based in systems theory offers an approach for combining policy and practice. Interactional family therapy incorporates the ecological perspective into the assessment and treatment process. An interactional approach to family therapy offers an alternative to family intervention for those practitioners frustrated by individual-based treatments.

This chapter concludes with an emerging practice approach, family health. The basic premises guiding family health are supported by extensive empirical research. Family health practice has a great deal to offer practitioners because it considers multiple factors in the assessment and treatment process. Bibliotherapy, an emerging practice approach consistent with the family health perspective is also offered in this chapter. Finally, a number of clinical instruments are presented that will help practitioners improve assessment from a family health perspective. A multilevel approach to assessment and intervention in family health enhances children's rights.

Appendix

Organizations Focusing on Children's Rights

Administration for Children and Families
<www.acf.dhhs.gov>

The Administration for Children and Families is a division of the U.S. Department of Health and Human Services. This Web site provides technical information and statistical data in regards to welfare reform.

American Adoption Congress
<www.american-adoption-cong.org>

This Web site provides information on adoption. It also is involved in advocacy and legislation development for children of adoption.

American Humane Association
<www.americanhumane.org>

This nationally recognized organization, known primarily for work in the area of child protection, provides references to publications specific to families.

Center for Law & Social Policy
<www.clasp.org>

The focus of this national center is on law social and social policy. This center places particular emphasis on welfare and children's policy.

Child Abuse Prevention
<http://child-abuse.com/>

This site, sponsored by the National Clearinghouse on Child Abuse and Neglect Information, offers information on prevention-related issues, resources for communities planning prevention activities, special resources on such topics as shaken baby syndrome and maltreatment of children with disabilities, and information on emerging practices in abuse and neglect prevention.

Child Trends, Inc.
<www.childtrends.org>

A national nonprofit organization dedicated to research focused on children, youth, and families. This Web site offers comprehensive data on how welfare reform affects children.

Child Welfare Institute
<www.gocwi.org>

This center focuses on children's rights and child legislation. It is also involved in child advocacy.

Child Welfare League of America
<www.cwla.org>

This organization has a general child welfare site, with specific pages related to developments in family preservation and lists of topically related publications provided by the organization.

Children's Bureau, Administration for Children and Families,
U.S. Department of Health and Human Services
<www.acf.dhhs.gov/programs/cb>

Contains information on federal initiatives in foster care and adoption and statistics, child abuse and neglect, and other related social problems.

Children's Defense Fund
<www.childrensdefense.org/>

The Children's Defense Fund is committed to the well-being of children. This Web site provides information about children and welfare reform but focuses mainly on statistics related to the condition of children in the United States.

Children's Rights, Inc.
<http://www.childrensrights.org/>

The goal of this institute is to ensure that the child welfare system follows the laws affecting children's lives. These laws deal with child abuse and neglect and child welfare.

Family Support America
<www.familysupportamerica.org>

This site promotes family support as a nationally recognized movement. It provides information on program models, evaluation studies and designs, policy and advocacy initiatives, upcoming events, and publications and products.

Institute for Women Policy Research
<www.iwpr.org>

This institute was established to research policies that affect women; a portion of the Web site covers welfare reform and contains information on domestic violence, reproduction, education, and issues that affect women in relation to welfare reform. The site also provides an online forum to discuss welfare issues.

National Campaign to Prevent Teen Pregnancy
<www.teenpregnancy.org>

This organization is supported by private donations with a goal to reduce the teen pregnancy rate by one-third between 1996 and 2005. This site is a source of information for local campaigns directed at teenagers and communities and has extensive research and statistical reports available.

National Center for Children in Poverty (NCCP)

The NCCP promotes policies and programs that work to reduce child poverty. This Web site provides statistics about children, along with information on how welfare reform affects children.

National Child Care Information Center

This center is part of the Children's Bureau, U.S. Department of Health and Human Services. It disseminates child care information in response to requests from states.

National Child Welfare Resource Center for Family-Centered Practice
<www.cwresource.org>

This center helps child welfare agency managers and staff translate the tenets of the Adoption and Safe Families Act of 1997 into family-centered practices that ensure the well-being and permanent placement of children while meeting the needs of families. The center helps clients learn how to forge linkages among the child welfare system, other support systems for families, and the courts, especially in the areas of substance-abuse treatment and domestic violence.

National Child Welfare Resource Center on Legal and Judicial Issues
<http://nccanch.acf.hhs.gov/pubs/reslist/cbttan/rclji.cfm>

This center provides expertise to clients on legal aspects of child welfare, including court improvement, agency and court collaboration, timely decisions on termination of parental rights, nonadversarial case resolution, reasonable efforts requirements, legal representation of children, permanent guardianship, confidentiality, and other emerging child welfare concerns.

National Clearinghouse on Child Abuse and Neglect Information
<www.calib.com/nccanch>

This organization is a national resource for professionals seeking information on the prevention, identification, and treatment of child abuse and neglect, and related child welfare issues.

National Committee to Prevent Child Abuse
<www.childabuse.org>

This is the Web site of a national advocacy organization whose purpose is to prevent and reduce child maltreatment. The site has numerous resources for advocates, including information packets, publications of statistics and trends, and lists of local chapters.

National Fatherhood Initiative
<www.fatherhood.org>

This site engages in educational, public information, and technical assistance initiatives to encourage involved, responsible, committed fathers. It serves all demographic groups, including traditionally underserved and high-risk groups.

National Indian Child Welfare Association
<www.nicwa.org>

This site is a source of comprehensive information on American Indian child welfare.

National Resource Center for Family Centered Practice
<www.uiowa.edu/~nrcfcp/>

Located at the School of Social Work, University of Iowa, the center promotes family-centered, culturally responsive practice across human service systems. It offers online publications and other information on prevention and family support.

Prevent Child Abuse America
<www.preventchildabuse.org.>

The goals of this organization are building awareness, providing education, and inspiring hope to everyone involved in the effort to prevent abuse and neglect of children. This organization has chapters in thirty-nine states and provides them with leadership and support for local abuse-prevention campaigns. The Web site has materials and resources, particularly for public information initiatives.

Resource Center for Adolescent Pregnancy Prevention
<www.etr.org/recapp/>

This is an online resource for educators of pregnancy prevention programs.

Urban Institute: Assessing the New Federalism
<www.urban.org/>

The Urban Institute provides extensive information on social and economic issues. "Assessing the New Federalism" is the Urban Institute's project examining welfare reform. In addition to information about all aspects of welfare reform, the site offers thorough and extensive research related specifically to families and children. The Web site also has a database with information about the efforts of each state in addressing welfare reform.

Welfare Information Network
<www.welfareinfo.org>

The Welfare Information Network is a foundation-sponsored Web site with extensive information on all aspects of welfare reform, including policies regarding immigrants, child support, teenage parenting, welfare-to-work programs, TANF, domestic violence, and child welfare.

Welfare Information Network: Teen Parents
<www.ssc.wisc.edu/irp/wrr/teenparents.htm>

The Welfare Information Network offers up-to-date policy information on issues relating to welfare reform. A special section of its Web site is devoted to policies concerning teen pregnancy and parenthood.

Glossary

adoption: A family created by law rather than by procreation.

Adoption and Safe Families Act of 1997 (ASFA) P.L. 105-89 (amended significant provisions of the Adoption Assistance and Child Welfare Act of 1980): Presents the "reasonable efforts" that must be made by state social service agencies to terminate parental rights. Requires permanency planning hearings within twelve months of out-of-home placement and initiation of termination of parental rights proceeding when a child is in care for fifteen of the past twenty-two months, except if the child is with a relative.

Adoption Assistance and Child Welfare Act of 1980: National legislation that encourages states to develop and implement important protections for children, including case plans, periodic reviews, and information systems.

advocacy: Representing and defending the rights of individuals and groups through direct intervention.

Americans with Disabilities Act of 1990: National legislation with the goal of providing people with disabilities the same civil rights protections as provided to individuals on the basis of race, sex, national origin, and religion.

assessment: The process of making judgments about information derived from a client system.

assessment instruments: Clinical instruments designed to assess the functioning of clients systems at multiple levels.

battered child syndrome: An early term used to describe the maltreated child and the circumstances surrounding maltreatment.

best interest: A standard that conveys to decision makers that a child in question is a victim of environmental circumstances, is at risk, and needs better alternatives in life.

bibliotherapy: Bibliotherapy is a strategy to help clients, including children, deal with emotional and adjustment problems as well as basic developmental needs through the use of books.

biological parents: The child's parents of procreation. Biological parents are not necessarily the child's psychological parents.

***Brown v. Board of Education* (1954):** In this case the U.S. Supreme Court ruled that "separate but equal" facilities in education were inherently unequal. The case has served as the basis for integrating children with disabilities into public schools.

case advocacy: An approach to advocacy that focuses on individual cases such as a single child whose rights have been violated.

case management: Coordinating helping activities on behalf of a client or client group.

cause advocacy: An approach that seeks to redress collective issues through social change, such as creating or improving social policies.

Child Abuse Prevention and Treatment Act of 1974: This law requires states to meet basic federal standards on custody provisions, which include the granting of state child welfare agencies the power to remove children from families for up to three days if an agency believes the child is at risk. Prior to the passage of the Child Abuse Prevention and Treatment Act, states had variable standards in place for protecting children from maltreatment.

child liberationist: This worldview argues children are entitled to self-determination. They should also have the same rights as adults.

child neglect: Involves omissive actions or a pattern of omissive actions on part of the caregiver. These actions result in physical, educational, social, and psychological delays.

child physical abuse: Abuse that includes commissive actions or a pattern of commissive actions on the part of a caregiver that results in physical injury to the child.

child protectionist: A view that suggests parents and society should shield children from the realities of adulthood because these realities have the potential to be dangerous, unsettling, or corrupting if children are exposed to them.

child psychological abuse: Abuse that includes threatening, disparaging remarks by a caregiver or other adult.

child sexual abuse: Involves sexual actions involving a child in any way. This behavior may be performed by an individual other than the caregiver with or without the caregiver's knowledge.

children at risk: Children born to or residing in a family system confronted with significant problems. Problems include poverty, disability, and substance abuse. These kinds of problems increase the probability of child maltreatment.

children with special needs: Children of color, who have disabilities, or who are members of sibling groups; term used in reference to adoption.

Children's Health Insurance Program (CHIP): A federal policy enacted in 1997 that provides incentives to the states to expand Medicaid coverage to additional children.

court: Public tribunals existing at the local, state, and federal levels which are mandated to deal with offenses against the nation or state or with controversies among people.

court-appointed special advocates (CASA): A trained nonattorney volunteer who helps to ensure that a child's best interest in the child welfare system is realized. This role is very similar to the GAL.

courts: Legal institutions in which attorneys play the leading roles and make most of the decisions.

discrimination: Differential treatment of individuals or groups based on race, ethnicity, sex, disability, and other legally protected groups.

dispositional stage: A court hearing to consider evidence on the question of what plan would be in the best interest of a child.

ecological perspective: This perspective explains human behavior in the context of social systems and the environment. It is a holistic orientation to assessment and treatment that includes the individual, family, organizational setting, community, and the larger social ecology.

Education of All Handicapped Children Act of 1975: National legislation that ensures a child with a disability a free appropriate public education.

empowerment: A process to help others increase their personal or political powers so they can take action themselves to improve their lives.

family: A system of two or more interacting persons who are either related by ties of marriage, birth, adoption, or who have chosen to commit themselves to one another as a unit for the common purpose of promoting physical, mental, emotional, social, economic, cultural, and spiritual growth and development.

family health: A state of holistic well-being of the family system. Family health is manifested by the development of and continuous interaction among the physical, mental, emotional, social, economic, cultural, and spiritual dimensions of the family, which results in the holistic well-being of the family and its members.

family policy: Policies aimed at supporting families in the areas of economic, medical, and social supports.

food stamps: In-kind assistance program funded by the United States Department of Agriculture and designed to supplement the food-purchasing power of eligible low-income households.

foster care: Any living arrangement in which children live with people who act as substitute parents.

Foster Care Independence Act/John H. Chafee Foster Care Independence Program of 1999 (FCLV Chafee) P.L. 106-169 (replaced the former Title IV-E Independent Living Program): This policy provides flexible funding to states to develop and implement independent living services to remain in foster care until age eighteen. Provides funding for room and board to youth who have left care and are less than twenty-one years old and provides Medicaid coverage of former foster children through twenty-one years.

guardian ad litem (GAL): An adult individual appointed by a court to protect the best interest of a minor child in a specific legal action; it is not necessary for the GAL to be an attorney.

Hazelwood School District v. Kuhlmeir (**1988**): In this case the U.S. Supreme Court ruled that public schools can monitor and censor the expression of students in the public school system.

holistic: The functional relation between parts and wholes.

homelessness: Having no adequate, fixed, regular nighttime place of residence.

human rights philosophy: This orientation concludes that all people are entitled to basic rights and that these rights are affirmed or reaffirmed through judicial and legislative actions.

humanitarian philosophy: This worldview stresses that people have intrinsic worth and dignity.

in loco parentis: A legal doctrine that means an agent other than parents, for example the courts, can make decisions ordinarily within the province of parents.

In re Gault (**1967**): The U.S. Supreme Court in this case ruled that the juvenile court must provide detained juveniles with due process.

In re Winship (**1970**): In this case, Winship, a twelve-year-old boy, was charged with stealing. He was adjudicated delinquent and the Supreme Court held that the standard of proof in a delinquency case is "beyond a reasonable doubt," the same standard required in adult court.

The Indian Child Welfare Act of 1978 (ICWA) P.L. 95-608: Defines the term "Indian child." This policy mandates that tribes have exclusive jurisdiction over child welfare issues involving an Indian child. It provides specific procedures to ensure compliance by the states.

individual education program (IEP): This plan outlines the educational program and services the child is supposed to receive under the Individuals with Disabilities Education Act (IDEA).

Individuals with Disabilities Education Act (IDEA): The new title for the Education of All Handicapped Children Act of 1975.

in-home services: Services provided to assist families and children that have special needs to remain living together in their own homes. Services include homemaker, home health care, and day care.

interactional family therapy: Has been called the "strategic" or the "communication" approach. This approach emphasizes the family communication process, systems theory, and the ecological context shaping the family system.

jurisdictional hearing: A hearing during which a judge decides if the evidence collected by the protective services agency is sufficient to sustain an allegation of child abuse or neglect.

Juvenile Court: Courts structured to act in the best interest of children.

Juvenile Justice and Delinquency Prevention Act of 1974 (JJDPA) P.L. 93-415 as amended by P.L. 107-273 (2002): Separates juvenile offenders from adult offenders in detention and places status offenders in secure detention facilities only if they have violated a court order and secure detention is found to be the only way to contain them. Establishes the Office of Juvenile Justice and Delinquency Prevention (OJJDP) and requires compliance as a condition for states to receive federal funding for prevention and treatment services.

***Kent v. United States* (1966):** This case questioned whether or not the juvenile court could take legal actions without a hearing. The Supreme Court ruled that juveniles were entitled to a hearing when detailed by the juvenile court.

least detrimental available alternative: Under this standard, realistic available alternatives are considered that bring the least harm to the child.

least restrictive environment: This term means that schools must include students with disabilities in the general education program and may not remove a student from it unless students cannot benefit from being in that program, even after the provision of supplementary aids and services and necessary related services.

Medicaid: Title XIX of the Social Security Act, Medicaid is a federal program designed to provide health care to poor people, including children.

Medicare: Title XVIII of the Social Security Act, Medicare is a federal program designed to provide health care for the elderly and for persons with long-term disabilities.

minority status of children: This status means children and adolescents do not have the capacity to act responsibly because of their underdeveloped cognitive, intellectual, and social development capacities.

Multiethnic Placement Act of 1994 P.L. 103-382 as amended by the Interethnic Placement Provisions of 1996: This policy prohibits the delay or denial of foster home or adoption placement on the basis of race, color, or national origin of the child or the potential foster or adoptive parent.

multiple placements: The movement of a child from one foster home to the next. This movement creates a lack of continuity with adult caregivers in the child's life.

New Jersey v. T.L.O. **(1985):** In this case, the Supreme Court ruled that school searches are constitutional as long as there are reasonable grounds for suspecting that the search will turn up evidence that a student has violated a law or rules of a school.

The No Child Left Behind Act (NCLBA): This act was signed into law by President Bush on January 8, 2002. The act made the largest changes to the federal education assistance program, the Elementary and Secondary Education Act (ESEA) since the inception of ESEA. The goals of the act are to ensure the funds spent by the federal government improve student achievement, implement annual assessments in reading and math in grades three through eight, increase greater accountability of teachers and improve teacher training, and increase the focus on math and science in the classroom.

parens patriae: A legal doctrine that means the state has a general duty to protect all citizens, especially those incapable of protecting themselves, such as children.

Pennsylvania Association for Retarded Children (PARC) v. Commonwealth of Pennsylvania **(1972):** A federal court ruled in this case that children with intellectual disabilities were entitled to a public education. The case has historical significance because it is seen as the basis for the Education of All Handicapped Children Act in 1975.

permanent plan: A plan that helps children in foster care to live in families that offer continuity of care and the opportunity to establish lifetime relationships.

The Personal Responsibility and Work Act of 1996 (HR 3734): A major provision of HR 3734 is to move welfare policy and programs from the federal level to the state and local levels. Under this legislation Medicaid is no longer an entitlement program for low-income families and time limits have been placed on a number of general welfare programs.

petition: A request for the court to make a decision about a child that has been brought to the attention of the protective services agency.

***Planned Parenthood v. Danforth* (1976):** The U.S. Supreme Court in this case found that a blanket rule requiring all minors to get consent from parents to procure an abortion was unconstitutional.

pluralism: The character, climate, or practices of a heterogeneous society in which competing interest groups shape policies and programs.

poverty: The lack of resources to achieve a reasonable standard of living. More children than any other group in the United States live below the poverty level.

preparationists: A position arguing that children must learn through experience; this experience will help them to be better prepared for adulthood.

primary prevention: Policy and program efforts aimed at the elimination of the causes of social problems.

the principle of free appropriate public education (FAPE): This term means that schools must individualize education for each student with a disability, provide needed related services, engage in a fair process for determining what is appropriate for each student, and ensure that the student's education indeed confers a benefit.

the principle of nondiscriminatory evaluation: Socioeconomic status, language, and other factors need to be discounted and must not bias the evaluation of the student with a disability.

the principle of parent and student participation: This principle means that schools must structure decision-making processes in such a way that parents of students with disabilities have opportunities to affect meaningfully the education the students are receiving. A related principle of enhanced accountability to pupils and parents is moving in the direction of report cards related to individualized goals and educational programs.

the principle of procedural due process: This principle means that the school must provide certain kinds of information (notice and access to records) to students with disabilities, special protection when natural parents are unavailable (surrogate parents), and access to a fair hearing process.

the principle of zero reject: This principle means that each school-age person with a disability has the right to be educated in a system of free appropriate public education (FAPE).

Protective Services: Specialized services aimed at treating neglected, abused, exploited, or rejected children.

psychological parent: The adult caregiver with whom a child has bonded. The caregiver does not necessarily have to be the biological parent.

reasonable accommodation: Any modification or adjustment under the Americans with Disabilities Act (ADA) that allows a qualified person with a disability to participate in the larger society. For a student with a disability, a reasonable academic modification might be providing the child with a tutor.

Rehabilitation Act of 1973: The first major national civil rights legislation enacted protecting persons with disabilities. Public and private entities receiving a certain level of federal funding must follow the mandates of this law.

residential treatment: Settings for children that are often staffed by various professionals, including social workers. In this kind of practice setting, practitioners offer critical services to juveniles; the families of these children are also typically part of the treatment plan.

***Roe v. Wade* (1973):** In this case the Supreme Court granted a constitutional protection allowing women the right to choose abortion early in pregnancy and the right of the state to regulate the termination of pregnancy after viability of the fetus; that is, when the life of the unborn child may be continued indefinitely outside the womb by natural or artificial life-supportive systems.

secondary prevention: Early detection and intervention to prevent problems from becoming more debilitating.

Section 504: The component of the Rehabilitation Act of 1973 that requires program access for persons with disabilities. It prohibits discrimination on the basis of disability in any program or activity offered by an entity or institution receiving a certain level of federal funding.

social class: The stratification of individuals and groups according to their socioeconomic assets.

social welfare: A nation's system of programs and benefits designed to provide the social, economic, educational, and health needs critical to the maintenance of society.

social welfare policy: Organized efforts by societies to facilitate the well-being of their citizens. These efforts are typically focused on the prevention or alleviation of selected social problems.

special education: Educational services and programs designed to meet the needs of children with special needs.

system: A social unit such as the family that consists of interdependent, interacting parts.

systems theory: A core theoretical grounding of the ecological perspective is systems theory. It helps practitioners understand how the client system functions in the larger social ecology. As a theoretical approach, it moves practitioners from a reductionistic view of human behavior to one stressing wholeness as the key to understanding individual behavior.

Temporary Assistance for Needy Families (TANF): A program created under the Personal Responsibility and Work Opportunity Reconciliation Act of 1996. The program is designed to provide support to needy families and their children.

tertiary prevention: Policy and program efforts aimed at limiting the effects of a problem after it has become manifest.

theory: A way of organizing a set of facts to explain or predict events.

***Tinker v. Des Moines Independent Community School District* (1969):** In this case the U.S. Supreme Court ruled that high school students had a right to wear black armbands to school to protest the Vietnam War.

undue burden: Under the Americans with Disabilities Act (ADA) this legal concept is defined as a significant difficulty or expense that would result if a program or building was made accessible to a person with a disability.

utilitarian philosophy: The central theme of this view is that usefulness determines the value of a person or thing to society. The utilitarian philosophy is reflected in the requirement under the Americans with Disabilities Act (ADA) that accommodations must be reasonable; for example, schools must make reasonable modifications to assist children with disabilities only if they are not an undue burden to the school system.

voluntary mediation process: A requirement under the Individuals with Disabilities Education Act (IDEA) that requires that the state have a voluntary mediation process if parents disagree with the school district's handling of their child's special education needs.

Welfare reform: Reform made by policymakers and legislators aimed at an ineffective general welfare system.

Wisconsin v. Yoder **(1972):** The U.S. Supreme Court ruled in this case that Amish parents could remove their children from public school at age fourteen.

worldview: A comprehensive conception of the world from a special point of view.

References

Foreword

Pardeck, J. T. (1996). *Social work practice: An ecological approach.* Westport, CT: Auburn House.

Chapter 1

Aldrich, R. and Associates (1976). *Toward a national policy for children and families.* Washington, DC: National Academy of Sciences.

Berger, P. L. and Neuhaus, R. (1977). *To empower people: The role of mediating structures in public policy.* Washington, DC: The American Enterprise Institute for Public Policy Research.

Carnegie Council on Adolescent Development (1989). *Turning points: Preparing American youth for the 21st century.* Washington, DC: Carnegie Council on Adolescent Development.

Cherlin, A. J. (1988). *The changing American family and public policy.* Washington, DC: Urban Institute Press.

Chung, W. S. and Pardeck, J. T. (1997). Explorations in a proposed national family policy for children and families. *Adolescence, 32,* 429-436.

Court Appointed Special Advocates (1996). *Volunteer training manual.* Springfield, MO: Court Appointed Special Advocates.

Downs, S. W., Moore, E., McFadden, E. M., Michaud, E. J., and Costin, L. B. (2004). *Child welfare and family services: Policies and practice.* Boston, MA: Allyn and Bacon.

Duquette, D. N. and Ramsey, S. (1987). Representation of children in child abuse and neglect cases: An empirical look at what constitutes effective representation. *University of Michigan Journal of Law Reform, 20,* 341-408.

Gil, D. (1970). *Violence against children.* Cambridge, MA: Harvard University Press.

Goldstein, J., Freud, A., and Solnit, A. J. (1973). *Beyond the best interests of the child.* New York: The Free Press.

Hartman, A. (1984). *Working with adoptive families beyond placement.* New York: Child Welfare League of America.

Hawes, J. M. (1991). *The children's rights movement.* Boston, MA: Twayne Publishers.

Helfer, R. E. and Kempe, C. H. (Eds.) (1968). *The battered child*. Chicago, IL: University of Chicago Press.

In re Gault, 387 U.S. 1 (1967).

Kadushin, A. and Martin, J. (1988). *Child welfare services* (Fourth edition). New York: Macmillan Publishing Company.

Kain-Caudle, P. R. (1973). *Comparative social policy and social security*. New York: University Press.

Kamerman, S. and Kahn, A. (1976). Explorations in family policy. *Social Work, 21,* 181-186.

Karger, H. and Stoesz, D. (2001). *American social welfare policy: A pluralist approach* (Fourth edition). New York: Longman.

Kaufman, P. and Frase, M. J. (1990). *Dropout rates in the United States: 1989*. Washington, DC: U.S. Department of Education.

Keniston, K. and The Carnegie Council on Children (1977). *All our children*. New York: Harcourt Brace Jovanovich.

Kent v. United States, 383 U.S. 541 (1966).

McGowan, B. G. and Meezan, W. (1983). *Child welfare: Current dilemmas and future directions*. Itasca, IL: F. E. Peacock Publishers.

Mnookin, R. (1973). Foster care—In whose best interest? (1973). *Harvard Educational Review, 43,* 599-638.

Morrissey, P. A. (1993). *The educator's guide to the Americans with Disabilities Act*. Alexandria, VA: American Vocational Association.

National Commission on Children (1991). *Beyond rhetoric: A new American agenda for children and families*. Washington, DC: Government Office.

O'Hare, W., Mann, T., Porter, K., and Greenstein, R. (1990). *Real life poverty in America: Where the American public would set the poverty line*. Washington, DC: Population Reference Bureau, Inc. and the Center on Budget and Policy Priorities.

PARC v. Pennsylvania, 343 F. Supp. 279 (E.D. PA 1972).

Pardeck, J. T. (1990). An analysis of the deep social structure preventing the development of a national policy for children and families in the United States. *Early Child Development and Care, 57,* 23-30.

Pardeck, J. T. (Ed.) (2002). *Family health social work practice: A macro level approach*. Westport, CT: Auburn House.

Pardeck, J. T. and Pardeck, J. A. (1987). Bibliotherapy in foster care and adoption. *Child Welfare, LXVI,* 269-278.

Pardeck, J. T. and Pardeck, J. A. (1998). *Children in foster care and adoption*. Westport, CT: Greenwood Press.

Piven, F. and Cloward, R. (1971). *Regulating the poor: The functions of public welfare*. New York: Random House.

Rice, M. (1977). *American family policy: Content and context*. New York: Family Service Association of America.

Schorr, A. L. (1968). *Exploration in social policy*. New York: Basic Books.

Tropman, J. E. (1985). The "Catholic ethic" vs. the Protestant ethic: Catholic social services and the welfare state. *Social Thought, 12*, 13-22.

U.S. Department of Commerce, Bureau of the Census (1989). *Projections of the population of the United States No. 1018: Projections of the population in the United States by age, sex, and race.* Washington, DC: Government Printing Office.

U.S. Department of Commerce, Bureau of the Census (1990). *Current population reports No. 447: Household and family characteristics.* Washington, DC: Government Printing Office.

Westman, J. C. (1991). *Who speaks for the children: The handbook of individual and class advocacy.* Sarasota, FL: Professional Resource Exchange, Inc.

Zill, N. and Schoenborn, C.A. (1990). *Developmental, learning and emotional problems: Health of our nation's children, United States, 1988.* Hyattsville, MD: U.S. Department of Health and Human Services, National Center for Health Statistics.

Chapter 2

Costin, L. B., Stoesz, D., and Karger, H. J. (1997). *The politics of child abuse in America.* New York: Oxford University Press.

Downs, S. W., Moore, E., McFadden, E. M., Michaud, E. J., and Costin, L. B. (2004). *Child welfare and family services: Policies and practice.* Boston, MA: Allyn and Bacon.

Farson, R. (1974). *Birthrights.* New York: Macmillan.

Freeman, M. (1997). *The moral status of children: Essays on the rights of the child.* The Hague, The Netherlands: Kluwer Law International.

Goldstein, J., Freud, A., and Solnit, A. J. (1973). *Beyond the best interests of the child.* New York: The Free Press.

Hawes, J. M. (1991). *The children's rights movement.* Boston, MA: Twayne Publishers.

Holt, J. (1974). *Escape from childhood.* New York: Ballantine Books.

Kramer, D. T. (2004). *Legal rights of children.* Colorado Springs, CO: Shepard's/ McGraw-Hill.

Mnookin, R. (1973). Foster care—In whose best interest? *Harvard Educational Review, 43*, 599-638.

Palmore v. Sidotti, 466 U.S. 429, 433 (1984).

Pierce v. Society of Sisters, 268 U.S. 510 (1925).

Planned Parenthood v. Danforth, 428 U.S. 52, 96 S.Ct. 2831, 49 L.Ed 2d 788 (1976).

Steinberg, L. (1991). Developmental considerations in youth advocacy. In Westman, J. C. (Ed.). *Who speaks for the children: The handbook of individual and class advocacy.* Sarasota, FL: Professional Resource Exchange, Inc.

Westman, J. C. (1991). The legal rights of parents and children. In Westman, J. C. (Ed.). *Who speaks for the children: The handbook of individual and class advocacy.* Sarasota, FL: Professional Resource Exchange, Inc.
Wisconsin v. Yoder, 406 U.S. 205 (1972).

Chapter 3

Alexander, R. and Curtis, C. M. (1995). A critical review of strategies to reduce school violence. *Social Work in Education,* 17, 73-83.
Brown v. Board of Education, 347 U.S. 483 (1954).
Constable, R., Shirley, S, and Flynn, J. P. (1996). *School social work: Practice, policy, and research perspectives* (Fourth edition). Chicago, IL: Lyceum.
Donohue, E. (1999). School house hype: Kids' REAL risks. *Education Digest,* 64(6), 4, 7.
Downs, S. W., Moore, E., McFadden, E. M., Michaud, E. J., and Costin, L. B. (2004). *Child welfare and family services: Policies and practice.* Boston, MA: Allyn and Bacon.
Lunenburg, F. C. and Ornstein, A. C. (2004). *Educational administration—Concepts and practices* (Fourth edition). Pacific Grove, CA: Brooks/Cole.
Malaspina, A. (1998). *Children's rights.* San Diego, CA: Lucent Books, Inc.
Mills v. Board of Education, 348 F. Supp. 866 (D. DC 1972).
Morrissey, P. A. (1993). *The educator's guide to the Americans with Disabilities Act.* Alexandria, VA: American Vocational Association.
PARC v. Pennsylvania, 343 F. Supp. 279 (E.D. PA. 1972).
Pardeck, J. T. (1998). *Social work after the Americans with Disabilities Act: New challenges and opportunities for social services professionals.* Westport, CT: Auburn House.
Pardeck, J. T. (2001). An update on the Americans with Disabilities Act: Implications for health and human services delivery. *Journal of Health and Social Policy,* 13, 1-15.
Pardeck, J. T. and Chung, W. C. (1992). An analysis of the Americans with Disabilities Act. *Journal of Health and Social Policy,* 4(1), 47-56.
Tennessee v. Lane, 541 U.S. 509 2004.
Westman, J. C. (1991). *Who speaks for the children: The handbook of individual and class advocacy.* Sarasota, FL: Professional Resource Exchange, Inc.

Chapter 4

Bronfenbrenner, U. (1970). *Two worlds of childhood: U.S. and U.S.S.R.* New York: Russel Sage.
Child Care Law Center (1995). Child care and the Americans with Disabilities Act. *Child Care Information Exchange,* 11, pp. 81-84.

Downs, S. W., Moore, E., McFadden, E. M., Michaud, E. J., and Costin, L. B. (2004). *Child welfare and family services: Policies and practice.* Boston, MA: Allyn and Bacon.

Fersh, D. and Thomas, P. W. (1993). *Complying with the Americans with Disabilities Act.* Westport, CT: Quorum Books.

Gormley, W. T. (1990). Regulating Mister Rogers' neighborhood: The dilemmas of day care regulations. *Brookings Review,* 8, 1-10.

Habermas, J. (1972). Towards a theory of communicative competence. In H. P. Drietzel (Ed.), *Recent sociology* (Second edition) pp. 115-148. New York: MacMillan.

Karger, H. and Stoesz, D. (2001). *American social welfare policy: A pluralist approach* (Fourth edition). New York: Longman.

Pardeck, J. T. (1997). The Americans with Disabilities Act and child care programs. *Early Child Development and Care,* 138, 29-39.

Pardeck, J. T. (1998). *Social work after the Americans with Disabilities Act.* Westport, CT: Auburn House.

Pardeck, J. T. (Ed.) (2002). *Family health social work practice: A macro level approach.* Westport, CT: Auburn House.

Pardeck, J. T., Pardeck, J. A., and Murphy, J. W. (1987) The effects of day care: A critical analysis. *Early Child Development and Care,* 27, 29-39.

Shapiro, J. P. (1993). *No pity: People with disabilities forging a new civil rights movement.* New York: Times Books.

Westman, J. C. (1991). Who speaks for the children: The handbook of individual and class advocacy. Sarasota, FL: Professional Resource Exchange, Inc.

Chapter 5

Community Learning Center Division of Youth Services (1999). *Student handbook.* Springfield, MO: Community Learning Center Division of Youth Services.

Community Learning Center Division of Youth Services (2000). *Juvenile offender victim's resource.* Springfield, MO: Community Learning Center Division of Youth Services.

Crider, A. B., George, G. R., Kavanaugh, R. D., and Solomon, P. R. (1986). *Psychology.* Glenview IL: Scott, Foresman and Company.

Hawes, J. M. (1991). *The children's rights movement.* Boston, MA: Twayne Publishers.

Kirst-Ashman, K. K. and Hull, G. H., Jr. (1999). *Understanding generalist practice.* Chicago, IL: Nelson-Hall.

Loewenberg, L. M. (1977). *Fundamentals of social interventions.* New York: Columbia University.

Chapter 6

Bavolek, S. J. (1989). Assessing and treating high-risk parenting attitudes. In J. T. Pardeck (Ed.), *Child abuse and neglect: Theory, research, and practice* (pp. 97-110). New York: Gordon and Breach Science Publishers.

Costin, L. B., Stoesz, D., and Karger, H. J. (1997). *The politics of child abuse in America.* New York: Oxford University Press.

Downs, S. W., Moore, E., McFadden, E. M., Michaud, E. J., and Costin, L. B. (2004). *Child welfare and family services: Policies and practice.* Boston, MA: Allyn and Bacon.

Finkelhor, D. (1984). *Child sexual abuse: New theory and research.* New York: Free Press.

Garbarino, J. (1977). The human ecology of child maltreatment: A conceptual model for research. *Journal of Marriage and the Family, 39,* 721-727.

Garbarino, J. (1991). The context of child abuse and neglect assessment. In J. C. Westman (Ed.), *Who speaks for the children: The handbook of individual and class advocacy* (pp. 183-203). Sarasota, FL: Professional Resource Exchange, Inc.

Gladston, R. (1965). Observations of children who have been physically abused by their parents. *American Journal of Psychiatry, 122,* 440-443.

Goldstein, J., Freud, A., and Solnit, A. J. (1973). *Beyond the best interests of the child.* New York: The Free Press.

Hamilton, L. R. (1989). Variables associated with child maltreatment and implications for prevention and treatment. In J. T. Pardeck (Ed.), *Child abuse and neglect: Theory, research, and practice* (pp. 29-54). New York: Gordon and Breach Science Publishers.

Helfer, R. (1975). *Diagnostic process and treatment programs.* Washington, DC: U.S. Government Printing Office.

Howing, P. T., Wodarski, J. S., Gaudin, J. W., and Kurtz, P. D. (1989). Clinical assessment instruments in the treatment of child abuse and neglect. In J. T. Pardeck (Ed.), *Child abuse and neglect: Theory, research, and practice* (pp. 69-82). New York: Gordon and Breach Science Publishers.

Howze-Brown, D. (1988). Factors predictive of child maltreatment. *Early Child Development and Care, 31,* 43-54.

Kadushin, A. and Martin, J. (1988). *Child welfare services* (Fourth edition). New York: Macmillan Publishing Company.

Kempe, C. H., Silverman, F., Steele, B., Droegemueller, W., and Silver, H. (1962). The battered child syndrome. *Journal of the American Medical Association, 181,* 17-24.

Milner, J. S. (1986). *The child abuse potential inventory* (CAP) (Second edition). DeKalb, IL: Psytec.

Milner, J. S. (1989). Applications and limitations of the child abuse potential inventory. In J. T. Pardeck (Ed.), *Child abuse and neglect: Theory, research, and practice* (pp. 83-95). New York: Gordon and Breach Science Publishers.

Minuchin, S. (1967). *Families of the slum: Exploration of their structure and treatment*. New York: Basic Books.

Oates, R. K. (1989). Ecological perspectives on child maltreatment: Research and intervention. In J. T. Pardeck (Ed.), *Child abuse and neglect: Theory, research, and practice* (pp. 55-67). New York: Gordon and Breach Science Publishers.

Pardeck, J. T. (1988). Social treatment through an ecological approach. *Clinical Social Work Journal*, 16, 92-104.

Pardeck, J. T. (1989). Family therapy as a treatment approach to child maltreatment. In J. T. Pardeck (Ed.), *Child abuse and neglect: Theory, research, and practice* (pp. 149-155). New York: Gordon and Breach Science Publishers.

Pardeck, J. T. (Ed.) (2002). *Family health social work practice: A macro level approach*. Westport, CT: Auburn House.

Pardeck, J. T. and Pardeck, J. A. (1998). *Children in foster care and adoption*. Westport, CT: Greenwood Press.

Pardeck, J. T. and Rollinson, P. A. (2002). An exploration of violence among homeless women with emotional disabilities: Implications for practice and policy. *Journal of Social Work in Disability and Rehabilitation*, 2, 63-74.

Sameroff, A. (1975). Transactional models in early social relations. *Human Development*, 18, 65-79.

Schere, P. A. (1991). Intervention in child abuse and neglect. In J. C. Westman (Ed.), *Who speaks for the children: The handbook of individual and class advocacy* (pp. 205-220). Sarasota, FL: Professional Resource Exchange, Inc.

Schmitt, B. D. and Beezley, P. (1976). The long-term management of the child and family in child abuse and neglect. *Pediatric Annals*, 5, 165-176.

Steele, B. (1976). Violence within the family. In R. Helfer and C. Kempe (Eds.), *Child abuse and neglect: The family and the community* (pp. 3-23). Cambridge, Mass: Ballinger Publishing.

Steele, B. and Pollock, C. (1968). A psychiatric study of parents who abuse infants and children. In R. E. Helfer and C. H. Kempe (Eds.), *The battered child* (Second edition) (pp. 89-133). Chicago, IL: University of Chicago Press.

Vondra, J. I. and Toth, S. L. (1989). Ecological perspectives on child maltreatment: Research and intervention. In J. T. Pardeck (Ed.), *Child abuse and neglect: Theory, research, and practice* (pp. 9-27). New York: Gordon and Breach Science Publishers.

Waxman, L. and Hinderliter, S. (1996). *A status report on hunger and homelessness in American cities: 1996*. Washington, DC: U.S. Conference of Mayors.

Whitbeck, L. B. and Hoyt, D. R. (1999). *Nowhere to grow: Homeless and runaway adolescents and their families*. New York: Aldine de Gruyer.

Wiehe, V. R. (1989). Child abuse: An ecological perspective. In J. T. Pardeck (Ed.), *Child abuse and neglect: Theory, research, and practice*. New York: Gordon and Breach Science Publishers.

Young, L. (1964). *Wednesday's children: A study of child neglect and abuse.* New York: McGraw-Hill.

Zorza, J. (2002). *Violence against women: Law, prevention, protection, enforcement, treatment, health.* Kingston, NJ: Civic Research Institute.

Chapter 7

Alinsky, S. D. (1946). *Reveille for radicals.* Chicago: University of Chicago Press.

Children's Rights (2004). Protecting children who cannot protect themselves. Retrieved May 19, 2004 <http://www.childrensrights.org/>.

Lewis, E. (1992). Social change and citizen action: A philosophical exploration for modern social group work. *Social Work with Groups,* 14, 23-34.

McGowan, B. G. (1987). Advocacy. In A. Minahan (Ed.), *Encyclopedia of social work: Vol. 1* (Eighteenth edition) (pp. 89-95). Silver Spring, MD: National Association of Social Workers.

Miley, K. K., O'Melia, M., and DuBois, B. (1995). *Generalist social work practice: An empowering approach.* Boston: Allyn and Bacon.

Pardeck, J. T. (1988). Social treatment through an ecological approach. *Clinical Social Work,* 16, 92-104.

Pardeck, J. T. (1990). An analysis of the deep social structure preventing the development of a national policy for children and families in the United States. *Early Child Development and Care,* 57, 23-30.

Pardeck, J. T. (1996). *Social work practice: An ecological approach.* Westport: CT: Auburn House.

Pardeck, J. T. (1998). *Social work after the Americans with Disabilities Act: New challenges and opportunities for social services professionals.* Westport, CT: Auburn House.

Pardeck, J. T. (1999). Family health and family policy. In J. T. Pardeck and F. K. O. Yuen (Eds.), *Family health: A holistic approach to social work practice* (pp. 137-152). Westport, CT: Auburn House.

Piven, F. and Cloward, R. (1971). *Regulating the poor: The functions of public welfare.* New York: Random House.

Rees, S. (1991). *Achieving power: Practice and policy in social welfare.* North Sydney, Australia: Allen & Unwin.

Rice, M. (1977). *American family policy: Content and context.* New York: Family Service Association of America.

Schorr, A. L. (1968). *Exploration in social policy.* New York: Basic Books.

Tropman, J. E. (1985). The "Catholic ethic" vs. the Protestant ethic: Catholic social services and the welfare state. *Social Thought,* 12, 13-22.

VeneKlasen, L. and Miller, V. (2001). *The action guide for advocacy and citizen participation.* Washington, DC: The Asia Foundation.

Westman, J. C. (1991). *Who speaks for the children: The handbook of individual and class advocacy.* Sarasota, FL: Professional Resource Exchange, Inc.

Chapter 8

Abidin, R. R. (1986). *Parenting stress index manual.* Charlottesville, VA: Pediatric Psychology Press.

Achenbach, T. M. and Edelbrock, C. S. (1979). The child behavior profile: II. Boys aged 12-16 and girls aged 6-11 and 12-16. *Journal of Consulting and Clinical Psychology,* 47, 223-233.

Alpern, G. D., Boll, T. J., and Shearer, M. W. (1980). *The developmental profile II manual.* Aspen, CO: Psychological Development.

Baird, M. A. and Doherty, W. J. (1990). Risks and benefits of a family systems approach to medical care. *Family Medicine,* 22, 396-403.

Barrera, M., Jr., Sandler, I. N., and Ramsay, T. B. (1981). Preliminary development of a scale of social support: Studies on college students. *American Journal of Community Psychology,* 9, 435-447.

Bavolek, S. J. (1984). *Handbook for the Adult-Adolescent Parenting Inventory.* Schaumberg, IL: Family Development Associates.

Beck, A. T. (1967). *Depression: Clinical, experimental and theoretical aspects.* New York: Harper & Row.

Bienvenu, M. J. (1969). Measurement of parent-adolescent communication. *Family Coordinator,* 19, 117-121.

Birleson, P. (1981). The validity of depression disorders in childhood and the development of a self-rating scale: A research report. *Journal of Child Psychology and Psychiatry,* 22, 73-88.

Buri, J. R. (1991). Parental authority questionnaire. *Journal of Personality and Social Assessment,* 57, 110-119.

Caldwell, B. M. and Bradley, R. H. (1978). *Home observation for measurement of the environment.* Little Rock: University of Arkansas.

Campbell, T. (1986). Family's impact on health: A critical review and annotated bibliography. *Family Systems Medicine,* 4, 135-328.

Campis, L. K., Lyman, R. D., and Prentice-Dunn, S. (1986). The parental locus of control scale: Development and validation. *Journal of Clinical Child Psychiatry,* 15, 260-267.

Carter, E. A. and McGoldrick, M. (Eds.) (1988). *The changing family life cycle: A framework for family therapy.* New York: Gardner Press.

Coleman, M. and Ganong, L. H. (1990). The use of juvenile fiction and self-help books with stepfamilies. *Journal of Counseling and Development,* 68, 327-331.

Forehand, R. L. and McMahon, R. J. (1981). *Helping the noncompliant child: A clinician's guide to parent training.* New York: Guilford Press.

Griffin, B. (1984). *Special needs bibliography: Current books for/about children and young adults.* DeWitt, NY: Griffin.

Haley, J. (1977). *Problem-solving therapy*. San Francisco, CA: Jossey-Bass.

Harter, S. (1982). The perceived competence scale for children. *Child Development, 53*, 87-97.

Hendershot, G. E. and LeClere, F. B. (Eds.) (1993). *Family health: from data to policy*. Minneapolis, MN: National Council on Family Relations.

Honig, A. S., Caldwell, B. M., and Tannenbaum, J. A. (1973). Maternal behavior in verbal report and in laboratory observation: A methodological study. *Child Psychiatry and Human Development, 3*, 216-230.

Hudson, W. W. (1990). *The multi-problem screening inventory*. Tempe, AZ: WALMYR.

Hudson, W. W. (1992). *The WALMYR assessment scales scoring manual*. Tempe, AZ: WALMYR

Hudson, W. W. and McIntosh, S. R. (1981). The assessment of spouse abuse: Two quantifiable dimensions. *Journal of Marriage and the Family, 43*, 873-888.

Humphrey, L. L. (1982). Children's and teacher's perspectives on children's self-control: The development of two rating scales. *Journal of Consulting and Clinical Psychology, 50*, 624-633.

Jansson, B. S. (2005). The reluctant welfare state: American social welfare policies-past, present, and future (Fifth edition). Pacific Grove, CA: Brooks/Cole Publishing.

Jones, S. L. (1986). A reformulation of the interactional approach to family therapy. In Whall, A. L. (Ed.), *Family therapy theory for nursing: Four approaches* (pp. 95-125). East Norwalk, CT: Appleton-Century-Crofts.

Karger, H. and Stoesz, D. (2001). *American social welfare policy: A pluralist approach* (Fourth edition). New York: Longman.

Klein, W. C. (1992). Measuring caregiver attitude toward the provision of long-term care. *Journal of Social Service Research, 16*, 147-162.

Kovacs, M. (1981). Rating scales to assess depression in school-aged children. *Acta Paedopsychiatrica, 46*, 305-315.

Kurdek, L. A. and Berg, B. (1987). Children's beliefs about parental divorce scale: Psychometric characteristics and concurrent validity. *Journal of Consulting and Clinical Psychology, 55*, 712-718.

Lindblom, C. E. (1959). The science of "muddling through." *Public Administration Review, 19*, 79-88.

Lowman, J. (1980). Measurement of family affective structure. *Journal of Personality Assessment, 44*, 130-141.

Magura, A., Moses, B. S., and Jones, M. A. (1987). *Assessing risk and measuring change in families: The family risk scales*. Washington, DC: Child Welfare League of America.

Magura, S. and Moses, B. S. (1986). *Outcome measures for child welfare services: Theory and applications*. Washington, DC: Child Welfare League of America.

Mayer, J. and Filstead, W. J. (1979). The Adolescent Alcohol Involvement Scale: An instrument for measuring adolescents' use and mis-use of alcohol. *Journal of Studies in Alcohol, 40*, 291-300.

McCroskey, J., Nishimoto, R., and Subramanian, K. (1991). Assessment in family support programs: Initial reliability and validity testing of the Family Assessment Form. *Child Welfare,* 70(1), 19-33.

McCubbin, H. I. and Patterson, J. M. (1983). Stress: The Family Inventory of Life Events and Changes. In E. E. Filsinger (Ed.), *Marriage and family assessment: A sourcebook for family therapy* (pp. 275-297). Beverly Hills: Sage.

Meinert, R., Pardeck, J. T., and Kreuger, L. (2000). *Social work: Seeking relevancy in the twenty-first century.* Binghamton, NY: The Haworth Press.

Milner, J. S., Gold, R. G., Ayoub, C., and Jacewitz, M. M. (1984). Predictive validity of the Child Abuse Potential Inventory. *Journal of Consulting and Clinical Psychology,* 52, 879-884.

Minuchin, S. (1974). *Families and family therapy.* Cambridge, MA: Harvard University Press.

Minuchin, S. and Wiltwyck School for Boys (1967). *Families of the slums: An exploration of their structure and treatment.* New York: Basic Books.

Moody, M. T. and Limper, H. K. (1971). *Bibliotherapy: Methods and materials.* Chicago: American Library Association.

Nowicki, S. and Strickland, B. R. (1973). A locus of control scale for children. *Journal of Consulting and Clinical Psychology,* 40, 148-154.

Olson, D. H. (1986). Circumplex Model Seven: Validation studies and FACES III. *Family Process,* 25, 337-351.

Olson, D. H. and Tiesel, J. W. (1993). Assessment of family functioning. In G. E. Hendershot and F. B. LeClere (Eds.), *Family health: From data to policy* (pp. 76-97). Minneapolis, MN: National Council on Family Relations.

Orton, G. L. (1997). *Strategies for counseling with children and their parents.* Pacific Grove, CA: Brooks/Cole Publishing.

Pardeck, J. T. (1981). The current state and new direction of family therapy. *Family Therapy,* 8, 21-27.

Pardeck, J. T. (1982). Family policy: An ecological approach supporting family therapy. *Family Therapy,* 9, 163-165.

Pardeck, J. T. (1996). *Social work practice: An ecological approach.* Westport, CT: Auburn House.

Pardeck, J. T. (1999). Family health and family policy. In J. T. Pardeck and F. K. O. Yuen (Eds.), *Family health: A holistic approach to social work practice* (pp. 137-152). Westport, CT: Auburn House.

Pardeck, J. T. and Pardeck, J. A. (1983). Using bibliotherapy in clinical practice with children of separation and divorce. *Arete,* 8, 10-17.

Pardeck, J. T. and Pardeck, J. A. (1987). Using bibliotherapy to help children cope with the changing family. *Social Work in Education,* 9, 107-116.

Pardeck, J. T. and Pardeck, J. A. (1989). Bibliotherapy: A tool for helping preschool children deal with developmental change related to family relationships. *Early Child Development and Care,* 47, 107-129.

Pardeck, J. T. and Yuen, F. (1997). A family health approach to social work practice. *Family Therapy,* 24(2), 115-128.

Paulson, M., Afifi, A. A., Chaleff, A., Thomason, M. L., and Liu, V. Y. (1975). An MMPI scale for identifying "at risk" abusive parents. *Journal of Clinical Child Psychology,* 4, 22-24.

Polansky, N. A., Chalmers, M. A., Buttenwieser, E., and Williams, D. P. (1981). *Damaged parents: An anatomy of child neglect.* Chicago: University of Chicago Press.

Polansky, N. A., Gaudin, J. M., and Kilpatrick, A. C. (1992). The Maternal Characteristics Scale: A cross validation. *Child Welfare,* 71(3), 271-280.

Poresky, R. H. (1987). Environmental Assessment Index: Reliability, stability and validity of the long and short forms. *Educational and Psychological Measurements,* 47, 969-975.

Quay, H. C. (1977). Measuring dimensions of deviant behavior: The Behavior Problem Checklist. *Journal of Abnormal Child Psychology,* 5, 277-287.

Rahdert, E. R. (Ed.) (1991). *The adolescent assessment/referral system manual.* Washington, DC: United States Department of Health and Human Services.

Robinson, E. A. and Eyberg, S. M. (1981). The dyadic parent-child interaction coding system: Standardization and validation. *Journal of Counseling and Clinical Psychology,* 49, 245-250.

Rosenberg, M. (1979). *Conceiving the self.* New York: Basic Books.

Rudman, M. K., Gagne, K. D., and Bernstein, J. E. (1993). *Books to help children cope with separation and loss: An annotated bibliography.* New York: R. R. Bowker.

Satir, V. (1967). *Conjoint family therapy.* Palo Alto, CA: Science and Behavior Books.

Shrodes, C. (1949). Bibliotherapy: A theoretical and clinical study. Doctoral dissertation, University of California, Berkeley.

Shrodes, C. (1961). The dynamics of reading: Implications for bibliotherapy. *ETC: A Review of General Semantics,* 18, 21-33.

Snyder, D. K. (1983). Clinical and research applications of the Marital Satisfaction Inventory. In E. E. Filsinger (Ed.), *Marriage and family assessment: A sourcebook for family therapy* (pp. 169-198). Beverly Hills: Sage.

Spanier, G. B. and Filsinger, E. E. (1983). The Dyadic Adjustment Scale. In E. E. Filsinger (Ed.), *Marriage and family assessment: A sourcebook for family therapy* (pp. 155-168). Beverly Hills: Sage.

Stonebrink, S. (1988). A measure of co-dependency and the impact of socio-cultural characteristics. Unpublished master's thesis, University of Hawaii School of Social Work.

Straus, M. A. (1979). Measuring intrafamily conflict and violence: The Conflict Tactics (CT) Scales. *Journal of Marriage and the Family,* 41, 75-88.

Timasheff, N. S. (1967). *Sociological theory: Its nature and growth.* New York: Random House.

Turner, R. J., Frankel, B. G., and Levin, D. M. (1983). Social support: Conceptualization, measurement, and implications for mental health. *Research in Community Mental Health,* 3, 67-111.

Vaux, A., Riedel, S., and Stewart, D. (1987). Modes of social support: The Social Support Behaviors (SS-B) Scale. *American Journal of Community Psychology,* 15, 209-237.

Wahler, R. G., House, A. E., and Stambaugh, E. E. (1976). *Ecological assessment of child problem behavior.* New York: Pergamon Press.

Whall, A. L. (Ed.) (1986). *Family therapy theory for nursing: Four approaches.* East Norwalk, CT: Appleton-Century-Crofts.

Wodarski, J. S. (1981). *The role of research in clinical practice: A practical approach for the human services.* Baltimore: University Park Press.

Yuen, K. O. and Pardeck, J. T. (1999). A family health approach to social work practice. In J. T. Pardeck and K. O. Yuen, (Eds.), *Family health: A holistic approach to social work practice* (pp. 101-114). Westport, CT: Auburn House.

Zaccaria, J. and Moses, H. (1968). *Facilitating human development through reading: The use of bibliotherapy in teaching and counseling.* Champaign, IL: Stipes.

Zatz, S. and Chassing, L. (1983). Cognitions of test-anxious children. *Journal of Consulting and Clinical Psychology,* 51, 526-534.

Index

Page numbers followed by the letter "f" indicate figures; those followed by the letter "t" indicate tables.

Order a copy of this book with this form or online at:
http://www.haworthpress.com/store/product.asp?sku=5533

CHILDREN'S RIGHTS
Policy and Practice, Second Edition

_____ in hardbound at $39.95 (ISBN-13: 978-0-7890-2811-2; ISBN-10: 0-7890-2811-5)

_____ in softbound at $29.95 (ISBN-13: 978-0-7890-2812-9; ISBN-10: 0-7890-2812-3)

Or order online and use special offer code HEC25 in the shopping cart.

COST OF BOOKS_____

☐ **BILL ME LATER:** (Bill-me option is good on US/Canada/Mexico orders only; not good to jobbers, wholesalers, or subscription agencies.)

☐ Check here if billing address is different from shipping address and attach purchase order and billing address information.

POSTAGE & HANDLING_____
(US: $4.00 for first book & $1.50 for each additional book)
(Outside US: $5.00 for first book & $2.00 for each additional book)

Signature_____

SUBTOTAL_____

☐ **PAYMENT ENCLOSED: $_____**

IN CANADA: ADD 7% GST_____

☐ **PLEASE CHARGE TO MY CREDIT CARD.**

STATE TAX_____
(NJ, NY, OH, MN, CA, IL, IN, PA, & SD residents, add appropriate local sales tax)

☐ Visa ☐ MasterCard ☐ AmEx ☐ Discover
☐ Diner's Club ☐ Eurocard ☐ JCB

Account # _____

FINAL TOTAL_____
(If paying in Canadian funds, convert using the current exchange rate, UNESCO coupons welcome)

Exp. Date_____

Signature_____

Prices in US dollars and subject to change without notice.

NAME_____

INSTITUTION_____

ADDRESS_____

CITY_____

STATE/ZIP_____

COUNTRY_____ COUNTY (NY residents only)_____

TEL_____ FAX_____

E-MAIL_____

May we use your e-mail address for confirmations and other types of information? ☐ Yes ☐ No
We appreciate receiving your e-mail address and fax number. Haworth would like to e-mail or fax special discount offers to you, as a preferred customer. **We will never share, rent, or exchange your e-mail address or fax number.** We regard such actions as an invasion of your privacy.

Order From Your Local Bookstore or Directly From
The Haworth Press, Inc.
10 Alice Street, Binghamton, New York 13904-1580 • USA
TELEPHONE: 1-800-HAWORTH (1-800-429-6784) / Outside US/Canada: (607) 722-5857
FAX: 1-800-895-0582 / Outside US/Canada: (607) 771-0012
E-mail to: orders@haworthpress.com

For orders outside US and Canada, you may wish to order through your local
sales representative, distributor, or bookseller.
For information, see http://haworthpress.com/distributors

(Discounts are available for individual orders in US and Canada only, not booksellers/distributors.)
PLEASE PHOTOCOPY THIS FORM FOR YOUR PERSONAL USE.
http://www.HaworthPress.com